T0226679

Necklift

Editor

MALCOLM D. PAUL

CLINICS IN PLASTIC SURGERY

www.plasticsurgery.theclinics.com

January 2014 • Volume 41 • Number 1

ELSEVIER

ELSEVIER

1600 John F. Kennedy Boulevard ● Suite 1800 ● Philadelphia, Pennsylvania, 19103-2899

http://www.theclinics.com

CLINICS IN PLASTIC SURGERY Volume 41, Number 1
January 2014 ISSN 0094-1298, ISBN-13: 978-0-323-22737-7

Editor: Joanne Husovski
Development Editor: Susan Showalter

© 2014 Elsevier Inc. All rights reserved.

This periodical and the individual contributions contained in it are protected under copyright by Elsevier, and the following terms and conditions apply to their use:

Photocopying
Single photocopies of single articles may be made for personal use as allowed by national copyright laws. Permission of the Publisher and payment of a fee is required for all other photocopying, including multiple or systematic copying, copying for advertising or promotional purposes, resale, and all forms of document delivery. Special rates are available for educational institutions that wish to make photocopies for non-profit educational classroom use. For information on how to seek permission visit www.elsevier.com/permissions or call: (+44) 1865 843830 (UK)/(+1) 215 239 3804 (USA).

Derivative Works
Subscribers may reproduce tables of contents or prepare lists of articles including abstracts for internal circulation within their institutions. Permission of the Publisher is required for resale or distribution outside the institution. Permission of the Publisher is required for all other derivative works, including compilations and translations (please consult www.elsevier.com/permissions).

Electronic Storage or Usage
Permission of the Publisher is required to store or use electronically any material contained in this periodical, including any article or part of an article (please consult www.elsevier.com/permissions). Except as outlined above, no part of this publication may be reproduced, stored in a retrieval system or transmitted in any form or by any means, electronic, mechanical, photocopying, recording or otherwise, without prior written permission of the Publisher.

Notice
No responsibility is assumed by the Publisher for any injury and/or damage to persons or property as a matter of products liability, negligence or otherwise, or from any use or operation of any methods, products, instructions or ideas contained in the material herein. Because of rapid advances in the medical sciences, in particular, independent verification of diagnoses and drug dosages should be made.

Although all advertising material is expected to conform to ethical (medical) standards, inclusion in this publication does not constitute a guarantee or endorsement of the quality or value of such product or of the claims made of it by its manufacturer.

Clinics in Plastic Surgery (ISSN 0094-1298) is published quarterly by Elsevier Inc., 360 Park Avenue South, New York, NY 10010-1710. Months of issue are January, April, July, and October. Business and Editorial Offices: 1600 John F. Kennedy Blvd., Suite 1800, Philadelphia, PA 19103-2899. Periodicals postage paid at New York, NY and additional mailing offices. Subscription prices are $490.00 per year for US individuals, $716.00 per year for US institutions, $240.00 per year for US students and residents, $555.00 per year for Canadian individuals, $853.00 per year for Canadian institutions, $630.00 per year for international individuals, $853.00 per year for international institutions, and $305.00 per year for Canadian and foreign students/residents. To receive student/resident rate, orders must be accompanied by name of affiliated institution, date of term, and the *signature* of program/residency coordinator on institution letterhead. Orders will be billed at individual rate until proof of status is received. Foreign air speed delivery is included in all *Clinics* subscription prices. All prices are subject to change without notice. **POSTMASTER:** Send address changes to *Clinics in Plastic Surgery*, Elsevier Health Sciences Division, Subscription Customer Service, 3251 Riverport Lane, Maryland Heights, MO 63043. **Customer Service: 1-800-654-2452 (US and Canada). From outside of the United States and Canada, call 314-447-8871. Fax: 314-447-8029. E-mail: JournalsCustomerService-usa@elsevier.com (for print support); JournalsOnlineSupport-usa@ elsevier.com (for online support).**

Reprints. For copies of 100 or more of articles in this publication, please contact the Commercial Reprints Department, Elsevier Inc., 360 Park Avenue South, New York, New York 10010-1710. Tel.: +1-212-633-3874; Fax: +1-212-633-3820; E-mail: reprints@elsevier.com.

Clinics in Plastic Surgery is covered in *Current Contents, EMBASE/Excerpta Medica, Science Citation Index, MEDLINE/ PubMed (Index Medicus), ASCA, and ISI/BIOMED.*

Printed and bound by CPI Group (UK) Ltd, Croydon, CR0 4YY

Transferred to digital print 2012

Contributors

EDITOR

MALCOLM D. PAUL, MD
Clinical Professor of Surgery, Aesthetic and
Plastic Surgery Institute, University of
California, Irvine, Newport Beach, California

AUTHORS

JOSE HORACIO ABOUDIB, MD
Professor and Chief, Plastic Surgery Service,
University of the State of Rio De Janeiro, Rio De
Janeiro, Brazil

ATHANASIOS ATHANASIOU, MD, PhD
Private Practice, Glyfada, Greece

ANTÔNIA MÁRCIA CUPELLO, MD
Staff, Plastic Surgery Service, University of
the State of Rio De Janeiro, Rio De Janeiro,
Brazil

CLAUDIO CARDOSO DE CASTRO, MD
Professor, Plastic Surgery Service, University
of the State of Rio De Janeiro, Rio De Janeiro,
Brazil

URMEN DESAI, MD, MPH
Associate Plastic Surgeon, Beverly Hills Body,
Los Angeles, California

RICHARD ELLENBOGEN, MD, FACS
Director Post Graduate Aesthetic Surgery
Fellowship Program; CEO Beverly Hills Body
Institute, Beverly Hills, California

DILSON LUZ, MD
Member, Brazilian Society of Plastic Surgery
and International Society Aesthetic Plastic
Surgery (ISAPS), Boa Viagem, Recife,
Pernambuco, Brazil

VINCENT C. GIAMPAPA, MD, FACS
Associate Clinical Professor, Division of Plastic
and Reconstructive Surgery, Rutgers
University, Newark, New Jersey

JEAN-PHILIPPE GIOT, MD
Division of Plastic Surgery, Department of
Surgery, Centre Hospitalier de l'Université
deMontréal, Montréal, Canada

RAUL GONZALEZ, MD
Associate Professor, Department of Surgery,
Medicine School of UNAERP, Universidade de
Ribeirao Preto, Ribeirão Preto, São Paulo,
Brazil

DARRYL HODGKINSON, MD, FRCS(C), FACS
Double Bay Day Surgery, The Cosmetic and
Restorative Surgery Clinic, Double Bay,
Sidney, Australia

JOHN H. JOSEPH, MD
Assistant Clinical Professor, Department of
Head and Neck Surgery, University of
California, Los Angeles, Los Angeles; Director,
Clinical Testing Center of Beverly Hills, Beverly
Hills, California

EMIL J. KOHAN, MD
Resident Physician, Aesthetic and Plastic
Surgery Institute, University of California -
Irvine Medical Center, Orange, California

DANIEL LABBÉ, MD
Private Practice, Caen, France

ALAN MATARASSO, MD, FACS
Plastic Surgery, Manhattan Eye, Ear and Throat
Hospital, Lenox Hill Hospital, North Shore-
Long Island Jewish Health System, New York,
New York

JOHN M. MESA, MD
Instructor in Plastic Surgery, Division of Plastic
Surgery, University of Alabama at Birmingham,
Birmingham, Alabama; Private Practice
Aesthetic, Plastic, Reconstructive and
Craniofacial Surgeon, Plastic Surgery Center
Internationale, Montclair, New Jersey

R. STEPHEN MULHOLLAND, MD, FRCS(C)
Private Aesthetic Plastic Surgery Practice,
Toronto, Ontario, Canada

MALCOLM D. PAUL, MD
Clinical Professor of Surgery, Aesthetic and
Plastic Surgery Institute, University of
California, Irvine, Newport Beach, California

OSCAR M. RAMIREZ, MD, FACS
Private Practice, "Ramirez Plastic Surgery" at
Elite Center for Cosmetic Surgery, Weston,
Florida; Private Practice, Clinica Corporacion
de Cirujanos Plasticos, Lima, Peru

GEORGIOS REMPELOS, MD
Private Practice, Athens, Greece

BRUNNO RISTOW, MD, FACS
California Pacific Medical Center,
San Francisco, California

ANA CLAUDIA ROXO, MD
Staff, Plastic Surgery Service, University of
the State of Rio De Janeiro, Rio De Janeiro,
Brazil

PATRICK TREVIDIC, MD
Plastic Surgeon, Scientific Director of
Expert2expert, Paris, France

GARRETT A. WIRTH, MD, MS, FACS
Associate Clinical Professor of Plastic Surgery,
Aesthetic and Plastic Surgery Institute,
University of California - Irvine Medical Center,
Orange, California

Contents

author has obtained improved cutaneous detachment; reduced postoperative swelling, edema, and ecchymosis; prophylaxis of facial nerve damage; and/or late postoperative hematoma formation.

the simplicity of the procedure, it has other advantages over medial plication of the muscle, because it is an incisionless procedure and requires less undermining that when using medial plication. The procedure has other advantages that are discussed this article.

The author presents his procedure for neck rejuvenation using a modified Fogli approach, which involves a transverse incision in Loré's fascia in the pretragal region, a "take-down" of the auriculoplatysmal ligament by resection to the body of the platysma where it crosses the sternomastoid muscle and then a triple cable suture fixation to the cut edge of Loré's fascia. Platysma bands are assessed for their degree of redundancy and those judged excessive in thickness or descent are resected via a submental incision. A strong, permanent elevation of the middle and the lower third of the platysma is achieved.

The first step is to assess the right candidate for this procedure. Then I select the type of incision depending on the candidate. In the Operative room, I always begin with extensive liposuction to include the jowl above the platysma and between the anterior platysma's bands, ceasing the liposuction at the mandibular line. I never perform fat resection. Then I follow with surgery which includes undermining the anterior border of the platysma and I perform a corset platysmarraphy with a barbed suture up to the superior border of the thyroid cartilage.

Isolated surgery of the neck without a facelift is increasingly in demand and a satisfying option for patients concerned with the aging appearance of the neck. It seems to be requested frequently in men and women and in patients who are satisfied with nonsurgical rejuvenation of the midface or who want to avoid preauricular scars of a facelift operation. Currently, neck surgery probably represents what *upper facelift surgery* meant to the earlier generation before nonsurgical alternatives were available to treat the midface. A variety of procedures are available from neck liposuction to submentalplasty or a neck lift.

Correction of aesthetic and anatomic deformities of the neck due to aging is a complex proposition, and the planning and approach depends on the findings during your initial examination. More than any area of the body, an in-depth knowledge of the anatomy is mandatory. The surgery can be very simple or highly technical, depending of your findings and surgical proposition. Surgeons should have in their armamentarium all the available surgical techniques to provide the best aesthetic result. Deep cervicoplasty is not for the occasional facial rejuvenative surgeon. You require experience in diagnosing neck problems, executing the proper surgical maneuvers, and effectively tackling acute and late complications if they occur.

CLINICS IN PLASTIC SURGERY

RELATED INTEREST

Neck Lift
Minimally Invasive Neck Lifts: Have they Replaced Neck Lift Surgery?
Steven H. Dayan, John P. Arkins, and Rahman Chaudhry
Facial Plastic Surgery Clinics of North America
Volume 21, Issue 2, May 2013
Theda C. Kontis, *Editor*

DOWNLOAD Free App!
Review Articles THE CLINICS

NOW AVAILABLE FOR YOUR iPhone and iPad

CLINICS IN PLASTIC SURGERY

FORTHCOMING ISSUES

Cleft Lip and Palate: Current Surgical Management
Thomas A. Imahara, MD, and
Jeffrey R. Marcus, MD, Editors

**Hand Problems in Plastic Surgery:
Simple and Complex**
Jin Bo Tang, MD, and
Michael Neumeister, MD, Editors

Body Contouring
Peter Rubin, MD, Editor

RECENT ISSUES

July 2013
Outpatient Plastic Surgery
Geoffrey R. Keyes, MD, and
Robert Singer, MD, Editors

April 2013
Outcomes Measures in Plastic Surgery
Kevin C. Chung, MD, MS, and
Andrea L. Pusic, MD, MHS, FRCSC, FACS, Editors

January 2013
Brow and Upper Eyelid Surgery:
Multispecialty Approach
Babak Azizzadeh, MD, and
Guy Massry, MD, Editors

RELATED INTEREST

June 2013
Minimally Invasive Wrist & Elbow Arthroscopy Meniscus Ankle and Surgeons
Steven H. Dayan, John P. Arkins, and Raphael Nabhan Chaudhry
Facial Plastic Surgery Clinics of North America
Volume 21, Issue 2, May 2013
Theda C. Kontis, Editor

NOW AVAILABLE FOR YOUR iPhone and iPad

Preface
The Neck: A Complex Cylinder

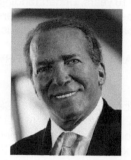

Malcolm D. Paul, MD, FACS
Editor

Cosmetic medical and surgical approaches to the aging neck have evolved over the past several decades and include noninvasive, minimally invasive, and open surgical approaches. Reviewing the history of the surgical approach to the aging neck revealed that early attempts at skin-only tightening were replaced with the aggressive approaches to the platysma muscles and principally preplatysmal fat removal in the 1960s and 1970s. Less aggressive platysma transection and repositioning as well as compartmental closed and open fat resection followed. Partial resection of the submaxillary glands and the anterior belly of the digastrics muscles was described as an option in further contouring the neck.

Although the approach to the upper and principally the middle third of the aging face has evolved to the appreciation of the need to address both volumetric and vector-based changes, surgical options in rejuvenating the neck have been mainly subtraction of skin, fat, gland, and muscle and repositioning of skin and platysma muscles. Assessing the aging neck begins with the observation of the cutaneous covering of the neck from the mandibular border to the clavicles. The next task is to understand the basic structure of the neck and its contents. The geometry of the neck is a simple cylinder. However, this cylinder is not hollow and therein lies the requirement for a template of procedures to address the anatomy hidden beneath the skin of this cylinder.

This issue of *Clinics in Plastic Surgery* examines many of the relevant options in rejuvenating the aging neck. Beginning with a thorough description of the clinical anatomy of the neck with an emphasis on correlating anatomy to procedure risks, this edition continues with

1. Topical treatments for improving the aging skin.
2. Advances in noninvasive and minimally invasive technologies using various injectables and energy sources to improve the quality of the skin envelope and tighten the collagen fibers within the dermis and within the fibrous septae between the superficial cervical fascia and the skin.
3. A techniques article to detail a range of open surgical procedures that address all of the internal components of the aging neck. There will be some overlap to the middle third of the face as some techniques utilize the continuity of the SMAS with the superior fibers of the platysma muscles to rejuvenate the neck by repositioning the SMAS and platysma as one or multiple flaps.

Authors for this issue were provided with a series of questions asking how they work with different types of anatomy in doing neck lifts. Each author either followed the question-and-answer format or provided a very brief, succinct description of their approach(es) and outcomes on their specific surgical technique(s), focusing on how they do it and why in order to offer surgeons options to help them assess their own surgical procedures and results. Not unexpectedly, there are many ways to approach the anatomical changes that one encounters in the aging neck. The authors describe their techniques from minimal access approaches to recontouring the neck

Clin Plastic Surg 41 (2014) xi–xii
http://dx.doi.org/10.1016/j.cps.2013.10.002
0094-1298/14/$ – see front matter © 2014 Elsevier Inc. All rights reserved.

to classical wide dissections from multiple access incisions, with both extremes describing their management of lax skin, compartmental lipodystrophies, platysma muscle bands, and their approach to the submaxillary gland and anterior belly of the digastrics muscles. Since it is mandatory that every option have a risk: reward ratio that clearly favors the reward(s), each author has been asked to describe the frequency of sequelae and complications that they have encountered and how they have been managed.

My goal in suggesting this topic to the publisher of *Clinics in Plastic Surgery* was to provide current safe and predictable options in cosmetic medical and surgical solutions for the aging neck. Of course, the public interest over the past several years in less invasive procedures with a faster recovery, allowing a quicker return to work and social obligations, must be judged with an eye toward providing a *meaningful, sustainable* solution to the aging neck. Certainly, some patients will be satisfied with a maintenance program with small steps while others will want a result that will last an average of 5 to 10 years. Understanding what our patients want has always been a cornerstone to having satisfied patients. Having said this, I believe that:

WHEN YOU BUY QUALITY, YOU ONLY CRY ONCE.

Malcolm D. Paul, MD, FACS
Aesthetic and Plastic Surgery Institute
University of California, Irvine
1401 Avocado Avenue, Suite 610
Newport Beach, CA 92660, USA

E-mail address:
mpaulmd@hotmail.com

Anatomy of the Neck

Emil J. Kohan, MD, Garrett A. Wirth, MD, MS*

KEYWORDS

- Neck anatomy • Plastic surgery • Neck lift

KEY POINTS

- Surgery of the neck is commonly performed by Plastic Surgeons.
- Neck anatomy and the location of important structures should be well known prior any neck surgery.
- Risks of complications are increased with secondary and tertiary surgeries.

Editor Commentary: Garrett Wirth was the first resident to rotate with me in the new plastic surgery training program at the Aesthetic and Plastic Surgery Institute at the University of California, Irvine. I asked him to write about neck anatomy because I knew that he would take a dry subject and bring it to life. His important contribution sets the stage for safely treating the aging neck by understanding what structures lie beneath the skin. The danger zones can be avoided after reading and digesting this important subject.

THE NECK AND ITS DIVISIONS

The neck is the region of the body between the clavicle and the mandible. If contains several vital structures (described later) and serves to separate the head from the torso. This discussion begins by describing the divisions of the neck and their contents. Subsequently, the layers of the neck are discussed and, finally, relevance with regards to surgery. Naturally, risks of complications are increased with secondary and tertiary surgeries.

Generally, the neck is clinically divided into an anterior triangle and posterior triangle. The anterior triangle of the neck is bordered by the following:

Anteriorly: the midline of the neck from the sternal notch to the chin
Posteriorly: the anterior margin of the sternocleidomastoid muscle
Superiorly: the mandible's inferior border

Anterior

The anterior triangle is further divided into 4 smaller triangles as follows:

Submental triangle (also known as suprahyoid triangle) is bordered by the hyoid bone inferiorly, anterior belly of the diagastric posterior/anteriorly, and the midline of the neck anteromedially. Its floor is formed by the mylohyoid muscle. This triangle contains submental lymph nodes and veins that subsequently join to form the anterior jugular veins. These veins are only at risk with very deep dissection; thus, injury is unlikely.

Submandibular triangle (also known as the digastric or submaxillary triangle) is bordered by the anterior and posterior bellies of the digastric muscle inferoanteriorly and inferoposteriorly, respectively. The superior aspect is bordered by the lower border of the mandible. This triangle contains the submandibular gland, facial vein and artery branches, and marginal mandibular branch of the facial nerve. The location of these structures deep to the platysma is significant during any neck operation. The location of the gland is relevant to any rejuvenation procedure involving the face/neck. The facial vein and artery must be protected for obvious reasons and damage to the marginal mandibular nerve has obvious deficits.

Carotid triangle (also known as the superior carotid triangle) is bordered by the anterior

Aesthetic and Plastic Surgery Institute, University of California - Irvine Medical Center, 200 S. Manchester Avenue, Ste 650, Orange, CA 92868, USA
* Corresponding author.
E-mail address: gwirth@uci.edu

Clin Plastic Surg 41 (2014) 1–6
http://dx.doi.org/10.1016/j.cps.2013.09.016
0094-1298/14/$ – see front matter © 2014 Elsevier Inc. All rights reserved.

border of the sternocleidomastoid posteriorly, superiorly by the posterior belly of the digastric and the stylohyoid muscle, and anteriorly by the omohyoid muscle. Its floor is formed by the middle and inferior pharyngeal constrictors, the hyoglossus, and the thyrohyoid. This triangle contains several important nerves, arteries, and veins. The nerves include branches of the facial nerve, cutaneous nerves, hypoglossal nerve, vagus nerve, sympathetic trunk, accessory nerve, and internal branch of the superior laryngeal nerve. The arteries include the superior aspect of the common carotid artery and its bifurcation into the external and internal carotids. The external carotid branches in this triangle include the superior thyroid artery, lingual artery, facial artery, occipital artery, and ascending pharyngeal artery. The veins contained in this space are the internal jugular vein (lateral to the common and internal carotid arteries) and corresponding veins to the external carotid artery—which drain into the internal jugular artery. This area is thus high risk, and great care has to be taken in this region with certain maneuvers.

Muscular triangle (also known as the inferior carotid triangle): this is bordered by the midline of the neck, the anterior aspect of the sternocleidomastoid posteriorly, and the superior belly of the omohyoid superoposteriorly. It contains supraclavicular nerve branches and the sternohyoid and sternothyroid muscles—which lie over the common carotid artery, the internal jugular vein, vagus nerve, branches of the ansa cervicalis, inferior thyroid artery, recurrent laryngeal nerve, sympathetic trunk and the esophagus, thyroid gland, and trachea medially.

Posterior

The posterior triangle of the neck is bordered by the following: anteriorly—posterior border of the sternocleidomastoid; posteriorly—anterior border of the trapezius; inferiorly—middle third of the clavicle; and apex—nuchal line of the occipital bone.

The posterior triangle of the neck is further divided into the following two triangles by the inferior belly of the omohyoid muscle: occipital triangle and subclavian triangle (or supraclavicular triangle). The posterior triangle of the neck contains several important nerves, muscles, vessels, and lymph nodes. These include

- Spinal accessory nerve
- Branches of the cervical plexus

- Roots and trunks of the brachial plexus
- Phrenic nerve
- Subclavian artery
- Transverse cervical artery
- External jugular vein
- Inferior belly of the omohyoid
- Scalene muscles
- Splenius muscle
- Levator scapulae muscle
- Occipital and supraclavicular lymph nodes

Dissection above this level is safe and dissection below should be carried out on the deep aspect of the muscle.

The neck, enclosed by skin and underlying fascia, has its fascia divided into superficial and deep cervical fascia.

The superficial fascia surrounds the platysma, cutaneous nerves, external and anterior jugular veins, and superficial lymph nodes. This is more important when performing neck lift surgery.

The deep cervical fascia (less critical for neck lift surgery) is further divided into the following 3 layers (all of which form the carotid sheath):

1. Investing layer: this surrounds the sternocleidomastoid and trapezius muscles and surrounds the entire neck posteriorly.
2. Pretracheal layer: this surrounds the viscera of the neck (trachea, thyroid gland, esophagus, pharynx, and larynx) and strap muscles.
3. Prevertebral layer: this surrounds the prevertebral muscles and forms a sheath for the brachial nerves and subclavian vessels.

THE MUSCLES OF THE NECK
The Platysma

The platysma is a thin sheet-like muscle that originates from the fascia over the pectoralis and deltoid below the clavicle **Figs. 1–3**. Superiorly, it inserts at the base of the mandible, orbicularis, and angle of the mouth. The blood supply consists of a dominant pedicle (a branch off of the submental artery) and a minor pedicle (branching off of the suprascapular artery). The platysma is innervated by the cervical branch of the facial nerve. It functions to draw inferiorly the corners of the mouth and lower the lower lip as well. The activity of the platysma can be deceptive as the mouth can move—thus, injuries to the marginal mandibular nerve should still be considered. When the teeth are clenched it pulls the skin of the neck superiorly. The anatomy of the platysma varies. There are 3 main categories of the anatomic platysma variation involving its decussation. Type I is the most common, occurring in 75% of patients—this involves decussation extending up to 2 cm below

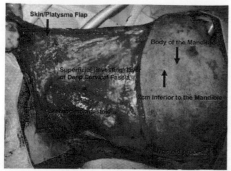
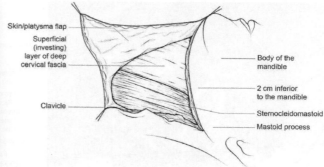

Fig. 1. Muscles of the neck.

the mandibular symphysis. Type II occurs in 15% of cases and the decussation is from the mandibular symphysis to the thyroid cartilage. Type III is having no decussations occurring—this occurs in approximately 10% of patients. The platysma is a significant contributor to the appearance of the aging neck; thus, reshaping of the platysma results in dramatic cosmetic changes. Multiple surgical techniques have been utilized to make cosmetic changes to the platysma. Many of these techniques will be discussed throughout this edition of Clinics in Plastic Surgery.

The Sternocleidomastoid

The sternocleidomastoid muscle originates from the sternal manubrium and medial aspect of the clavicle and attaches to the mastoid process of the temporal bone and superior nuchal line. It is supplied by the occipital artery and superior thyroid artery. It functions to flex the neck (when both sides are activated), extends the head, and rotates the head. It is also an accessory muscle of inspiration. The motor component of the muscle is from the accessory nerve and the sensory innervation is from the cervical plexus. The variation in this muscle is the extent of its origination off of

the clavicle, an attachment that may be as much as 7.5 cm. Dissections over this muscle posteriorly must be carried out with care to avoid the great auricular and spinal accessory nerves.

The Trapezius

The trapezius is a large muscle that originates in the occipital protuberance and medial superior nuchal line and attaches at the lateral third of the clavicle, acromion process, and spinous processes of C7-T12. It functions to shrug the shoulders (elevation of the scapulae) as well as to rotate, depress, and retract the scapulae. It is a significant component of maintaining posture and works with different muscle groups to allow throwing (with the deltoid) and various scapular movements (ie, with the serratus and rhomboids). The main motor component is supplied by the spinal accessory nerve (cranial nerve XI), and minor motor and sensory components are supplied by cervical spinal nerves C3 and C4. The main artery supplying the trapezius is the superficial branch of the transverse cervical artery, or the superficial cervical artery, and in 20% the subclavian artery. This is rarely of importance for correction of the neck, but the nerves are still at risk.

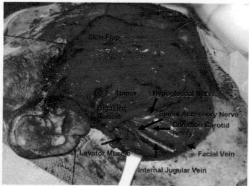
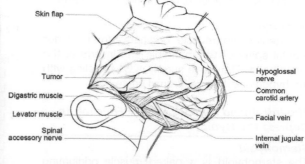

Fig. 2. Intraoperative neck anatomy.

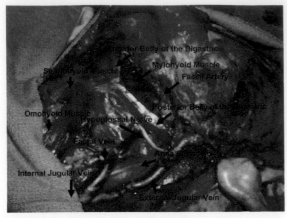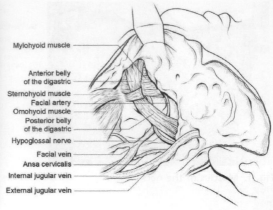

Fig. 3. Intraoperative neck anatomy.

The Suprahyoid Muscles (Which Function to Elevate the Hyoid)

Digastric

The digastric muscle is made up of an anterior belly, which originates from the digastric fossa in the inner surface of the mandible and attaches to the hyoid bone, and a posterior belly, which originates from the mastoid process of the temporal bone and attaches to the hyoid bone. The blood supply of the anterior belly is from the submental branch of the facial nerve and the blood supply of the posterior belly is from the occipital artery. The nerve supply of the anterior belly is a branch of the mandibular division of the trigeminal nerve (the mylohyoid nerve) and the posterior belly is supplied by the facial nerve. The anterior belly of the digastric muscle has been of significant interest to many plastic surgeons. Various dissection and surgical techniques are discussed throughout this edition of Clinics in Plastic Surgery.

Mylohyoid

The mylohyoid originates from the mylohyoid line of the mandible and attaches at the hyoid bone and median raphe. The nerve supply is a branch of the mandibular division of the trigeminal nerve (the mylohyoid nerve). The blood supply is from the mylohyoid branch of the inferior alveolar artery.

Geniohyoid

The geniohyoid muscle originates from inferior mental spine of the mandible and inserts at the hyoid bone. The nerve supply is C1 traveling with the hypoglossal nerve (cranial nerve XII).

The Infrahyoid Muscles (Which Function to Depress the Hyoid)

Sternohyoid

The sternohyoid is a paired muscle originating at the sternum and attaching at the hyoid. It is innervated by the ansa cervicalis (C1-C3) and the blood supply is from the superior thyroid artery.

Sternothyroid

The sternothyroid, wider and shorter in length than the sternohyoid, originates at the sternal manubrium and attaches at the thyroid cartilage. It is innervated by the ansa cervicalis (C1-C3) and the blood supply is from the superior thyroid artery.

Thyrohyoid

The thyrohyoid originates at the thyroid cartilage and attaches at the hyoid bone. It is innervated by C1 via the hypoglossal nerve and its blood supply is from the superior thyroid artery.

Omohyoid

The omohyoid originates from the scapula and attaches at the hyoid bone. It has 2 muscle bellies separated by a tendon. After arising from the scapula, it passes behind the sternocleidomastoid. Its tendon is surrounded and held in place by the deep cervical fascia. It is innervated by the ansa cervicalis (C1-C3).

THE LYMPH NODES

There are an estimated 300 lymph nodes in the neck. Several classification systems exist for cervical lymph nodes. The nodes are often classified by levels and/or regions as follows:

Classification by levels
    Level Ia: submental triangle
    Level Ib: submandibular triangle
    Level II: upper jugular nodes
    Level III: middle jugular nodes
    Level IV: lower jugular nodes
    Level V: posterior triangle nodes
    Level VI: anterior triangle nodes
    Level VII: upper mediastinal nodes

Classification of nodes by region
  Deep lymph nodes: submental and submandibular nodes
  Anterior deep cervical nodes: prelaryngeal, thyroid, pretracheal, and paratracheal nodes
  Deep cervical lymph nodes: lateral jugular, anterior jugular, and jugulodigastric nodes
  Inferior deep cervical lymph nodes: jugulomyoid and supraclavicular nodes

When operating on the neck, superficial lymph nodes are encountered (deep nodes are usually not encountered in aesthetic surgery). In general, they should not affect an operative plan, unless they seem abnormal. In the cases in which a lymph node seems abnormal, excisional biopsies should be performed and location of the node clearly documented. These lymph nodes are mostly encountered in the retroaurical and submental areas.

THE SUBMANDIBULAR GLAND

The submandibular glands are under each side of the mandible and above the digastric muscles—located in the submandibular triangle. They receive blood supply from branches of the facial artery. The mylohyoid muscle divides the submandibular gland into a superficial and deep portion. Medial to the submandibular gland are the mylohyoid and hyoglossus muscles as well as the lingual and hypoglossal nerves. Lateral to the gland are the platysma, mandible, and cervical branches of the facial nerve, which supplies the platysma and gives branches to the cervical cutaneous nerve. It is important to understand these relationships and possible variations before undergoing any resection. Superficial partial excisions are part of some aesthetic neck surgeries.

BLOOD SUPPLY OF THE NECK
Arteries

The neck and face are well-vascularized areas (see **Figs. 2** and **3**). The blood supply of the neck is based mainly on the external carotid artery and its branches. The external carotid artery, beginning at the upper border of the thyroid cartilage, gives off the superior thyroid artery, ascending pharyngeal artery, lingual artery, facial artery, and occipital artery (from inferior to superior) in the carotid triangle (described previously). Subsequently, it gives off the posterior auricular artery before forming its terminal branches, the maxillary artery, and superficial temporal artery. These are at risk with aggressive dissection but generally easy to identify.

The facial artery takes off superior to the lingual artery above the hyoid bone. It courses posterior to the submandibular gland along the medial aspect of the ramus of the mandible. It gives off the submental artery prior to running along the lower aspect of the mandible anterior to the masseter. It is important to note its location just underneath the platysma because it is here that it is intersected by the marginal mandibular nerve. It then curves toward the oral commissure. The facial artery subsequently becomes a major contributor to the facial soft tissues.

The submental artery (branching off of the facial artery) runs along the mylohyoid muscle below the body of the mandible. It then courses toward the chin and forms a network of arteries with the inferior labial and mental arteries.

The posterior auricular artery takes off just above the digastric muscle and courses between the ear and mastoid process. It divides into an auricular branch and occipital branch, which subsequently anastomoses with branches of the occipital artery branches. These are at risk during surgery but at low risk for complication.

Veins

The venous drainage system of the head and neck is made of an intricate network of vessels, knowledge of which is relevant to all facial and neck surgeries. This knowledge is required to avoid potential intraoperative and postoperative bleeding and edema and to avoid associated nerves and other structures. The veins of the neck are generally divided into a superficial and deep system.

Facial vein

The facial vein, after coursing through the face, crosses over the mandible and superficial to the submandibular gland and digastric muscle—coming to join the internal jugular vein posteriorly approximately at the level of the base of the mandible. The facial vein, along with all of the deep veins of the neck, drain into the internal jugular vein. These are generally not problematic during aesthetic surgery of the neck but more at risk with gland and digastric work.

Superficial veins

The superficial veins of the neck ultimately drain into the external jugular vein—which receives blood from the face and scalp. The external jugular vein is formed by the posterior facial vein and posterior auricular vein. It receives blood from several veins, including the posterior external jugular vein, transverse cervical vein, transverse scapular vein, anterior jugular vein, internal jugular vein, and, occasionally, the occipital vein. It begins in line with the angle of the mandible in the parotid gland and runs along the posterior aspect of the sterno-cleidomastoid until the clavicle, where it drains into the subclavian vein. The platysma lies on top of the external jugular vein—and the superior portion of the external jugular vein runs parallel with the great auricular nerve. Knowledge of this anatomy is imperative when dissecting deep to the platysma.

Anterior jugular veins

The anterior jugular veins are in the submandibular area and are formed by several smaller veins in the submaxillary region. These course along the medial aspect of the strap muscles superiorly toward the sternal notch until they drain into the external jugular vein or subclavian vein. Again, knowledge of this anatomy is imperative when dissecting deep to the platysma because there is a propensity toward bleeding.

SIGNIFICANT NERVES IN THE NECK
Great Auricular Nerve

The great auricular nerve provides sensory innervation to the skin over the parotid gland and mastoid process and parts of the ear (see **Figs. 2** and **3**). Made up of the second and third cervical nerves, the great auricular nerve comes around from the posterior aspect of the sternocleidomastoid and ascends up toward the parotid gland. Subsequently, it divides into anterior and posterior branches. Inferior to the ear it courses intimately with the external jugular vein. The great auricular nerve is the most likely nerve to be damaged during a facelift—this is at approximately 6.5 cm inferior to the tragus, where it courses over the sternocleidomastoid. Damage to this nerve may result in numbness to the aforementioned areas and potential neuroma development.

Cutaneous Cervical Nerve

The cutaneous cervical nerve (transverse cervical nerve or superficial cervical nerve) provides sensory innervation to the anterior and lateral aspects of the neck. Like the great auricular nerve, it too is

made up of the second and third cervical nerves. It also comes around the posterior aspect of the ster-nocleidomastoid (approximately in the middle part of the muscle) and courses over the muscle under the external jugular vein until it perforates the deep cervical fascia and divides into two branches, the ascending and descending branches—subsequently innervating the anterior and lateral aspects of the neck. This division into ascending and descending branches is deep to the platysma. The sternocleidomastoid muscle is the reference point for this nerve intraoperatively.

Greater Occipital Nerve

The posterior scalp is innervated by the greater occipital nerve—a branch of dorsal ramus of C2. This nerve comes through the suboccipital triangle, pierces the trapezius, and ascends to supply the scalp. The lesser occipital nerve arises from C2-3 (ventral ramus), courses along the posterior aspect of the sternocleidomastoid muscle, and ascends to supply the lateral aspects of the scalp posterior to the ear. These nerves are not usually problematic during aesthetic neck surgery.

Marginal Mandibular Nerve

The marginal mandibular nerve is a branch of cranial nerve VII (the facial nerve) and innervates muscles of the lower lip and chin. The muscles innervated by the marginal mandibular nerve include the depressor labii inferioris, the depressor anguli oris, and the mentalis. These muscles serve to depress the bottom lip, depress and move the corner of the mouth laterally, and protrude the lower lip, respectively. Knowledge of the course of the marginal mandibular nerve is important for surgeons. It follows the mandibular border as it courses laterally and anteriorly. It runs as low as 2 cm below the inferior border of the mandible prior to crossing the facial vessels. Thus, if dissecting deep to the platysma, it is imperative to remain at least 2 cm inferior to the mandible in this area to avoid damaging the marginal mandibular nerve.

Nonsurgical Neck Laxity Correction

John H. Joseph, MD[a,b,*]

KEYWORDS

- Neck • Neuromodulators • Dermal fillers • Nonsurgical • Laxity

KEY POINTS

- Surgery is still the optimal and most efficacious way to treat laxity in the neck.
- Neuromodulators and fillers play a limited role in addressing laxity in the neck.
- Energy based technologies such as Laser or Focused Ultrasound are getting better at correcting excess laxity of skin in the neck.

Editor Commentary: *In planning this issue of Clinics, I wanted to include all available options that would address the aging neck. Importantly, the aging of the skin envelope had to be addressed. I asked Dr Joseph to write this article. In so doing, he has summarized the available options and has informed us about the limitations of the various energy based skin tightening devices. I agree that we need to follow these technologies and see what we can expect as an average improvement realizing that patients show varying skin texture, collagen composition, elasticity and the effects of the environment on skin aging.*

INTRODUCTION

At present, there are many different modalities that can be used outside of surgery to treat the aging neck. That being said, nothing works as well as surgery to address the primary issue of laxity in the neck. Although excess laxity is the major reason patients seek treatment in the region of the neck, surgery is unable to resolve issues such as texture, dynamic lines of expression, and pigment problems.

The alternative nonsurgical choices available today to improve the neck can be broken down into 3 groups: neuromodulators (NMs), fillers, and energy-based technologies (EBT). Because noninvasive or minimally invasive procedures have exploded in popularity over the last 10 years, refinement in EBT has occurred for the treatment of neck skin laxity. Due to a demand for minimally or noninvasive treatments, device companies have spent considerable amounts of time and money to advance new technologies. Currently, for select patient populations, these forms of energy-based treatments are now beginning to show noticeable improvement in treating the condition of excess skin laxity of the neck.

NEUROMODULATORS

Neuromodulation of the neck can improve some components of the aging neck. In particular, the medial hyperdynamic platysmal bands, which project forward blunting the cervicomental angle, can often be dramatically improved from injection of a NM in select cases. It has been difficult to predict those patients who will benefit the most from this treatment. A trial injection is the only and best way to make this determination. The same can be done for the lateral bands. Some improvement in the jowl area can also be achieved by the judicious use of a NM on the

[a] Department of Head & Neck Surgery, University of California, Los Angeles, 757 Westwood Plaza, Los Angeles, CA 90095, USA; [b] Clinical Testing Center of Beverly Hills, 9400 Brighton Way, Suite 203, Beverly Hills, CA 90210, USA

* Clinical Testing Center of Beverly Hills, 9400 Brighton Way, Suite 203, Beverly Hills, CA 90210.

E-mail address: drjohnjoseph@sbcglobal.net

Clin Plastic Surg 41 (2014) 7–9

http://dx.doi.org/10.1016/j.cps.2013.09.007

0094-1298/14/$ – see front matter © 2014 Elsevier Inc. All rights reserved.

platysma, which overlies this area. By reducing the downward pull of the platysma on the jowl, some mild elevation can improve the jawline. This technique has been described as a "Nefertiti" lift. Occasionally, the treatment of necklace lines can be accomplished with the broad application of a NM to treat the platsyma muscle overall. Care must be exercised with this form of therapy to avoid adverse events from the spread of the NM to adjacent and deeper musculature of the neck.

DERMAL FILLERS

Fillers play a limited role in improving the appearance of the neck. Loss of volume seems not to play as large a role in the aging neck as in the mid face area. The reestablishment of the jaw line from the use of fillers in the pre- and postjowl region, along with the angle of the mandible, is of great benefit toward enhancing the patient's appearance. A "Witches Chin" deformity can be lessened by the proper placement of filler inferior to the problem area. Rarely a mild "Cobra Neck" deformity can be improved by using filler. Although these treatments do little to elevate lax skin, they improve the overall esthetic appearance of the neck without surgery.

ENERGY-BASED TECHNOLOGIES

EBT now offer the best form of nonsurgical treatment to combat neck laxity. There are 4 types of energy sources that can be used to tighten the neck:

1. Broad band light or intense pulsed light
2. Radiofrequency
3. Laser
4. Micro-focused ultrasound with visualization

Broad Band Light or Intense Pulsed Light

Broad band light or intense pulsed light was first used to treat acne and, as a byproduct, was also found to be advantageous for superficial dyschromias of the face and telangiectasia. After treatment of these aforementioned issues, the skin was noticeably improved in texture and, as a result, mild tightening was observed. Because of this result, technology companies attempted to investigate other energy sources to enhance the tightening seen with broad band light. The fundamental principle or mechanism of action on the skin is not exactly known. It is assumed the wound repair mechanisms are engaged, which result in collagen and elastin production and fibroblast replication.

Radiofrequency

The first devices were externally applied and RF based. Initially these devices had problems with efficacy because the treatments were very painful and the results were limited due to the excessive pain. As a result, the improvement was inconsistent and modest at best. An overall 10% to 20% improvement was obtained by a small number of subjects treated. As the parameters for the treatments were refined, so were the number of patients getting results, but an overall ceiling of 20% improvement seemed to be reached. Occasionally dramatic results were obtained in a very small number of patients but these rare cases could not be guaranteed to the patient as a realistic result.

Today, there are numerous devices that attempt to externally use RF to bulk heat the underlying dermis and subcutaneous tissues to address skin laxity. There is another device called Thermagen, which uses a subcutaneous probe to bulk heat the tissues. The technique is similar to liposuction, using a cannula-like probe that delivers RF at the tip. Although invasive, this technology may provide a way to avoid passing the energy through the skin and, instead, direct to the underlying tissues. Protocols to use this novel way to deliver the RF energy are currently in progress and may support US Food and Drug Administration clearance for this use in the future.

Laser

Lasers have also been used to tighten skin of the face and neck. Again, the exact mechanism of action is not known but the wound repair mechanism seems to be engaged in the process of tightening the skin. External skin resurfacing and chemical peels have always been found to tighten facial laxity and refurbish the texture and appearance of the skin. Although not used primarily for this benefit, phenol and fully ablative carbon dioxide skin resurfacing (FACDSR) do provide a noticeable degree of improvement on skin laxity. The down time and postprocedure aftermath of these treatments led companies to develop minimally ablative and nonablative ways to use lasers to address skin laxity. Fractionated CO_2 laser does improve skin laxity with less down time than phenol or FACDSR but still not as successfully as surgery. A 1064 Yag laser such as the one used by Alma on their Clear Lift procedure is an example of laser used to tighten the neck by passing the energy through the skin to the deeper layers. There are a multitude of laser frequencies and devices available today that attempt to tighten the face and neck with no downtime or superficial ablation of the skin. Over time, many of these devices and companies have come and gone because of inconsistencies of results and the overall limited improvement obtained.

Micro-Focused Ultrasound with Visualization

Micro-focused ultrasound by Ulthera is the latest device that uses this novel energy source to inflict a wound to the deeper layers of the skin and subcutaneous tissues while bypassing the surface of the skin. With a high degree of accuracy and precision the device allows the user to visualize the exact tissue layer where the energy is deposited. The specific targeting includes the SMAS layer. The micro-focused ultrasound creates linear rows of discrete thermal coagulation points. Initially the treatment was uncomfortable, and like other devices, the proper protocol and amounts of thermal coagulation points per treatment were not optimized. Since then, a significant refinement in the treatment protocol has resulted in a more reliable and efficacious result. This technology is the only EBT US Food and Drug Administration cleared to produce a "lift" of submental and neck tissue. A validated quantitative measure of neck lift has demonstrated a clinically significant result in 73% of patients. The degree of improvement was often seen to exceed the 20% ceiling of other technologies. Again these results are obtained when proper candidates are selected and a full treatment is performed. New protocols have reduced the pain from the procedure so patients are able to enjoy more consistent and noticeable improvement.

SUMMARY

In summary, to date no device or treatment with filler or NM has been developed yet that provides the degree and consistency in improving laxity of skin in the neck as surgery does. Attempts over the years to create nonsurgical and minimally or noninvasive treatments for neck laxity were initially poor at best. Fillers and NMs play a very limited role in correcting neck laxity. The most promise lies in energy-based devices, which initiate wound repair mechanisms. For the properly selected patient the current technologies are improving at providing a reasonable alternative to surgery. As these devices continue to evolve, there may come a day when surgery will be obsolete or play a greatly diminished role in correcting neck laxity. This day, however, appears to be further down the road more than many of us would like.

Nonexcisional, Minimally Invasive Rejuvenation of the Neck

R. Stephen Mulholland, MD, FRCS(C)

KEYWORDS

- Noninvasive neck rejuvenation • Laser neck procedures • Radiofrequency neck procedures
- Bodytite • NeckTite • FaceTite • Smartlipo • Fractora • Fractional CO2 • RF
- Radiofrequency skin resurfacing

KEY POINTS

- This paper describes nonexcisional techniques for neck rejuvenation.
- External and subcutaneous and subdermal laser, RF, light, ultrasound and injectable treatments are reviewed.

Editor Commentary: Steve and I have been involved in several emerging technologies and have had the pleasure to discuss alternative and additive modalities with him frequently. In this chapter, Steve takes us on the journey of minimally invasive and non-invasive energy based techniques to rejuvenate the aging neck. He frequently combines these techniques with open aggressive procedures. Realizing that minimally invasive techniques can provide measureable skin tightening has provided yet another opportunity to answer our patients' desires for procedures with a quicker recovery. Of course these can be stand alone procedures or performed along with or following more aggressive surgical maneuvers. The patient with minimal submental and or jowl laxity after a face and necklift looks to us to provide a solution. For sure, we enjoy surgery more than our patients and therein lies their quest for an easy answer without surgical expense and downtime.

INTRODUCTION

Western civilization is experiencing a "boom in boomers," an aging population, with population decline. The aging population in Western Europe, North America, and Asia has disposable income and the mantra of "youth and vitality" has this generation increasingly presenting for aesthetic treatments, specifically noninvasive or nonexcisional procedures.[1,2] The neck aesthetic subunit often ages early and more noticeably than other head and neck regions and is one of the most common motivations for patients to present to aesthetic physicians for rejuvenation options. The neck undergoes extrinsic and intrinsic aging changes in all anatomic layers and the aesthetic physician must be well equipped to deal with aging cervical concerns, both surgically and nonsurgically. For the surgeon, being skilled in nonsurgical cervical rejuvenation is critical, as many patients may opt for nonexcisional cervical enhancements, alone, or in combination with other facial cosmetic surgical procedures. For the cervical surgeon, a familiarity and expertise with nonsurgical management of the neck, as "stand-alone" therapy or as postoperative "protect your investment" treatments, may help extend and prolong the achievements achieved surgically.

A youthful neck is most often characterized by an acute cervicomental angle and a firm, well-defined jawline (**Fig. 1**). The skin in a youthful neck is smooth and devoid of horizontal or vertical neck lines; has no platysmal bands; no visible submandibular glands; small, nonhypertrophic masseter

---

Private Aesthetic Plastic Surgery Practice, SpaMedica 66 Avenue, Toronto, Ontario M5R 3N8, Canada
E-mail addresses: mulhollandmd@spamedica.com; sy@spamedica.com

Clin Plastic Surg 41 (2014) 11–31
http://dx.doi.org/10.1016/j.cps.2013.09.002
0094-1298/14/$ – see front matter
© 2014 Elsevier Inc. All rights reserved.

Ideal youthful neck

- acute cervicomental angle
- defined jawline
- smooth, even, bright skin
- no horizontal or vertical lines
- no platysmal bands
- no visible submandibular glands
- non-hypertrophic masseter muscles
- Minimal melanin or vascular lesions

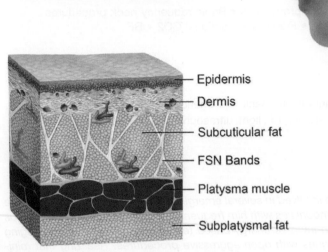

Epidermis

Dermis

Subcuticular fat

FSN Bands

Platysma muscle

Subplatysmal fat

Fig. 1. Characteristics of an ideal youthful neck.

muscles; and skin that is bright and even in color, with minimal melanin or vascular lesions.[3]

For the nonexcisional cervical physician, aesthetic rejuvenation of the neck with a multimodal, nonexcisional, minimally invasive approach will be a very common and popular component of the facial aesthetic practice. For all aesthetic physicians, familiarity with the aging tissue changes of the neck, its anatomy and the possible minimally invasive, nonexcisional interventions, including laser, light, radio frequency, high-intensity focused ultrasound (HIFU) energy-based therapy, both transepidermal and subdermal approaches, injectable soft tissue fillers, neuromodulators, and ablative and nonablative technologies for skin rejuvenation, as well as suture-based suspensory techniques, all used alone or in combination, will be a valuable asset to the global aesthetic head and neck cosmetic physician.

This article brings together the "tried-and-true" nonexcisional neck rejuvenation methodologies, which have had long-term, peer-reviewed success in the literature, together with procedures and technologies that have emerged in the past few years that have proven to be successful and complementary. It is my hope that this information assists aesthetic physicians in enhancing their global approach to nonexcisional rejuvenation of the neck.

AESTHETIC CERVICAL ANATOMY OF THE NECK

This issue of *Clinics in Plastic Surgery* deals extensively with the surgical options and management of the aging neck. However, the noninvasive, minimally invasive and nonexcisional solutions for the neck are often what patients opt for and, many times, are techniques and strategies that can also enhance and/or extend surgical results, or can be applied following surgical neck procedures to provide smaller enhancements and maintenance of the outcome postoperatively.

The aesthetic anatomy of the neck can be divided into several layers, from superficial to deep, starting with the skin, subcutaneous tissue, superficial musculo-facial layer and deep subplatysmal structures (**Fig. 1**).[3] In this section, the relevant anatomy of the neck as it pertains to minimally invasive and noninvasive rejuvenation procedures is outlined and then cervical enhancement options for each layer follow.

The anatomic classification of the neck pertains to the aging structures as the patient sees them and to the anatomic options and targets that the aesthetic physician may elect to treat, which are outlined in **Fig. 2**.

Cutaneous Cervical Layer

The cutaneous layer of the neck consists of a relatively thin epidermis and dermis. The skin of the neck is subject to multiple mimetic and cervical animations, and tensile and compressive loads. Bending the neck in the anterior-posterior direction, as well as side to side with active contraction of the underlying platysma, can lead to horizontal lines or "necklace lines." The skin ages as a consequence of intrinsic (genetic) and extrinsic (applied) forces. The neck itself is often exposed to the sun and may not be protected by sunscreen and, thus, often presents with significant extrinsic photoaging. Cervical photoaging will result in increased epidermal thickness, degeneration of functional elements of the cervical dermis, such as useful collagen, elastin, and ground substances, with accumulation of whorls of elastotic collagen in the deep dermis (**Fig. 3**). Aging laxity of the platysmal muscle may lead to visible central and/or lateral neck bands. The

cumulative photoaging of the neck combined with intrinsic aging and mimetic changes results in a typical aging cutaneous cervical envelope, characterized by thin "crepe" skin, diffuse dyschromia and telangiectasia, with multiple vertical lines in the midline, affectionately termed "iguana neck," as well as horizontal lines, centrally and laterally, attributed to platysma and cervical motion (see **Fig. 3**).

The aesthetic physician needs to be especially skilled in the rejuvenation of the cutaneous layer of the neck. Surgeons performing excisional neck surgery can often fail to deliver optimal neck rejuvenation results by not being familiar with, or equipped to deal with, superficial aging changes of the neck. The superficial cutaneous aging changes to the neck do not respond optimally to pure tensile repositioning characterized by neck lift surgery, but rather, respond to multimodal, noninvasive treatments designed to improve the more superficial color, tone, and texture of the skin. Similarly, nonsurgical aesthetic physicians need to familiarize themselves with the various nonexcisional treatment modalities used to rejuvenate the cutaneous layers of the aging neck.

Aging changes in the neck

- Obtuse cervicomental angle
- Poorly-defined jawline
- Photo-aging changes in the skin
- Horizontal or vertical lines due to platysmal and cervical motion
- Central and lateral neck bands
- Visible submandibular glands
- Hypertrophic masseter muscles

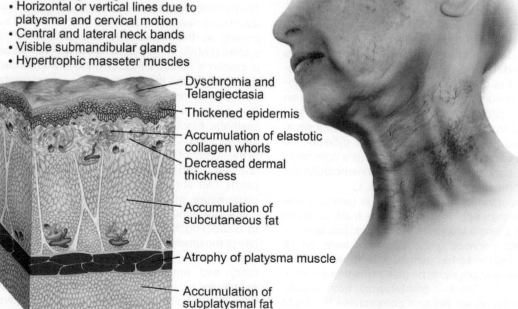

Dyschromia and Telangiectasia
Thickened epidermis
Accumulation of elastotic collagen whorls
Decreased dermal thickness
Accumulation of subcutaneous fat
Atrophy of platysma muscle
Accumulation of subplatysmal fat

Fig. 2. Anatomic classification of the neck pertaining to the aging structures and to the anatomic options with potential for treatment.

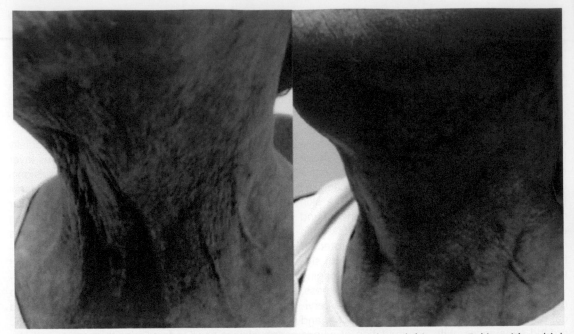

Fig. 3. (*Left*) Cervical photoaging resulting in laxity of the platysmal muscle and thin "crepe" skin, with multiple vertical lines and horizontal lines attributed to platysma and cervical motion. (*Right*) Complete cervical dyschromia correction combined with décolleté provides a natural blend between the rejuvenated neck, the chest, and the face.

Subcutaneous Cervical Layer

Deep to the cutaneous, epidermal-dermal layer of the neck is subcutaneous or adipose tissue. There can be a wide variation in aging presentations of the cervical subcutaneous layer. Some patients have aging cervical phenotypes that have little subcutaneous fat between the deep dermis and the underlying platysma, whereas other patients have extensive amounts of subcutaneous fat between the dermis and the platysma. Modest-to-large amounts of subcutaneous fat will create an obtuse angle to the cervicomental angle and detract from what is considered a youthful neck. An ideal neck consists of a vertical cylinder, the trachea and muscles that connect as a right angle to the floor of the mouth and submandibular tissue, forming a 90° angle (see **Fig. 1**).

Subcutaneous fat of the neck is generally less fibrous than adipose tissue of the trunk or thighs and is a single layer with interlobular fascial components connecting the platysma layer on its deep surface to the dermis. It is imperative that the aesthetic physician be able to diagnose subcutaneous fat, which is preplatysmal, from subplatysmal fat, which will also compromise the acute cervicomental angle, but is more difficult to access and to treat without incisional or excisional surgery.

The Cervical Platysmal Layer

The platysma bands are wide, broad strap-shaped skeletal muscles extending from the clavicle to the dermal attachments along the mandibular border.[3] The cervical platysma is invested by the superficial layer of the deep cervical fascia and will extend superiorly as the superficial-muscular aponeurotic system (SMAS).[3] The platysma comes in a number of anatomic variants, including those with no central diastasis and those with a wide central diastasis that may present as medial platysmal bands. The platysma itself has been attributed the aesthetic function of a secondary depressor of the modiolus, synergetic to the primary depressor of the corner of the mouth, the depressor angularis oris (DAO), and in this fashion, the lateral platysmal bands can act as a depressor of the midface, commissure, mouth, and jawline.[4,5]

The platysma itself, when hypertonic, can lead to distracting aesthetic contours, causing obliquity of the otherwise youthful, acute cervicomental angle (see **Fig. 3**). With aging and muscle flaccidity and atrophy, the platysma bands can contribute to cervical laxity, creating a loose, adynamic, and obtuse neck. The aesthetic physician should be prepared to treat the cervical platysma when it is aesthetically important to the an optimal rejuvenative outcome, and excisional physicians, in addition to surgical manipulation and excision transection techniques, must also be able to manage nonoperatively any dynamic preoperative and postoperative cervical aesthetic problems.

Subplatysmal Aesthetic Structures

The subplatysmal aesthetic structures that can be treated nonexcisionally or minimally invasively include the densely packed, subplatysmal, adipose tissue that is present in a significant proportion of cervical aesthetic patients, as well as the submandibular glands. The deeply compacted subplatysmal fat lies on top of the mylo-hyoid muscle and may contribute to a "double chin" or obtuse cervicomental angles, and the aesthetic physician needs to be able to diagnose, either by clinical examination or ultrasound techniques, when the submental fat is due to preplatysmal or subplatysmal pathology. Suctioning subplatysmal fat may require a small incisional localization of the platysma to place the cannula in the subplatysmal plane, or open subplatysma lipectomy.

The other deep platysmal structures that occasionally require aesthetic management and nonexcisional treatment are the submandibular glands. The submandibular glands measure approximately 3×5 cm and are secondary salivary glands that rest in the lateral floor of the mouth and they can occasionally be visible as lumps or soft tissue shadows in the lateral neck. These glands can be particularly visible postoperatively after tightening or suction reduction procedures of the anterior and lateral neck. Both the excisional and nonexcisional cervical aesthetic physician needs to be able to address prominent submandibular glands (see **Fig. 3**).

ANATOMIC, NONEXCISIONAL MANAGEMENT OF THE NECK
Cutaneous Layer

Chromaphore-based pathologies
Melanin-dyschromia Melanin discoloration, or dyschromia, of the neck is common, given its sun-exposed location on the head and neck region. Commonly patients will neglect to apply sunscreen or sunblock on their cervical region, yet cover the backs of their hands and their face. Over years of sun exposure, the typical photoaging appears. Melanin and dyschromia lesions can range from isolated solar lentigines or diffuse dyschromia and melisma. Diffuse brown discoloration is a very common presentation of the aging neck. Quite frequently, the dyschromia is associated with other signs of photoaging, including thickening and hyperkeratosis of the epidermis layer, thinning dermis

with decreased elasticity, decreased functional elastin and collagen, and elastotic whorls of disorganized collagen in the deep reticular dermis associated with fine or deep cervical rhytides (see **Figs. 2 and 3**). The cervical skin will often look vertically fissured or, even further, cobblestoned Fitzpatrick VIII, IX, or X type of rhytids can appear (see **Figs. 2 and 3**). The dyschromia, with or without photoaging is best treated with modalities that are either specific to the discoloration or nonspecific and ablative in nature. Historically, chemical peels of the neck, like complete laser ablative resurfacing, were fraught with potential for wound-healing complications, as the adnexal tissue in the cervical dermis is limited, with few sebaceous glands, pilosebaceous units, eccrine, or apocrine glands to *reepithelialize completely ablated skin*.[6,7] Hence, the use of moderate strength office or home-based topical chemical correction of cervical dyschromia has become popular, with very mild chemical peels or "bleaching agents."[8,9] The bleaching regimens generally consist of combinations of retinoic acids 0.05% to 0.1%, or tazarotene 0.025% to 0.01%, alone or combined with hydroquinone 4%, 6%, or 8%, 4% Kogic acids, and occasionally mild hydrocortisone-compounded substances. Prescriptive skin bleaching programs include the popular Tri-Luma. Other skin care regimens, such as Obagi, SkinCeuticals, Physician Choice of Arizona, Skin Medica, and others, have been quite popular in gradually bleaching dyschromia of the neck using home-based programs. Office-based treatments include stronger chemical peels, although the risk of delayed *reepithelialization* and hypopigmentation or hyperpigmentation is greater when stronger preparations of glycolic, glycolic acid, trichloroacetic acid, or stronger topical chemical ablatives are deployed.

Over the past 15 years, chromophore-based lasers and light-based sources have become the mainstay of skin color correction and are arguably the gold standard of dyschromia-associated aging of the neck. Chromophore-based lasers and light-based systems have wavelengths of light that are specifically attracted to intra-epidermal, epidermal-dermal, and superficial dermal melanin, through a process called selective photothermolysis.[10] Typically, wavelengths in the range of 500 to 800 nm will have some increased affinity for and selective absorption of superficial cervical melanin-based concerns. Some of the monochromatic focal wavelengths for the improvement of superficial epidermal-dermal melanin include the 532-nm wavelength Potassium titanyl phosphate (KTP) lasers, 694.5 nm Q-switched Ruby, and the 755 long-pulsed or Q-switched Alexandrite lasers, which have all been deployed in specific correction of dyschromia of the neck.[11–13] Pulsed dye lasers in the 585-nm wavelength have also been deployed to treat not only vascular lesions but pigmented lesions of the neck.[12] However, the one most popular light-based rejuvenation of the neck for dyschromia and vascular chromophores has become intense pulsed light, or IPL.[14,15] IPL, broad-band flash lamps, or xenon flash lamps consist of visible wavelengths of light from 500 nm to 1200 nm all released during the same pulse. Specific cutoff filters are deployed in a variety of methods, with or without direct water cooling, interpositional gel, or air cooling in a multitude of intense pulsed light systems available on the market to treat very effectively melanin and vascular discoloration of the cervical skin. Generally, for cervical rejuvenation in skin types I, II, and III, with dyschromia, cutoff filters in the 515-nm to 580-nm range have been very successful.[14,15] For skin types 4 and 5, long wavelength cutoff filters in the 590-nm to 640-nm ranges, lower energies, and longer pulse configurations have allowed the treatment of darker discoloration in patients with more advanced Fitzpatrick skin type.[16] Using gentle energy with broad melanin absorption coefficients and overlapping 20% or so, each pulse can provide safe, effective clearance for even the most severe cervical dyschromia over several sessions.

Intense pulsed light treatments of the neck usually require 1 treatment every 3 to 4 weeks for a total of 3 to 5 treatments. It can be quite common to cause striping in the neck following early IPL therapy in patients with extensive photoaging, which is caused by a combination of aggressive settings and not overlapping the light guide sufficiently during each treatment, which results in aggressive fading of the treated neck adjacent to untreated skin that does not fade in color. Gentle settings, multiple sessions, and overlapping or crisscrossing can avoid this problem. It is important that the IPL settings are gentle moderate in fluence, as IPL may induce a permanent hypopigmentation or discoloration of the skin.[13–15] Monochromatic treatment of the neck with focal monochromatic laser systems can cause a reticulated hypopigmented appearance to the cervical skin.[13]

It is common in dyschromia and photoaging of the skin to have a relative white and protected area of skin color immediately under the chin and submentum superior to the hyoid cartilage. This "white patch" represents the shaded area naturally created by the projected pogonion of the mandible. It is important to try to blend the "white under chin" into the more dyschromic and photoaged, lateral, and inferior aspects of the neck. It is also important to blend the discoloration of the central and lateral neck into the posterior triangle and trapezius border. Additionally, carrying the treatment over the clavicle onto the precordial region will help minimize risk of demarcation between a treated neck and an untreated décolleté. Often, combining complete cervical dyschromia correction with décolleté will provide a natural blend between the rejuvenated neck, the chest, and the face (see **Fig. 3**).

The recent addition of fractional nonablative, fractional ablative lasers, and ablative fractional radiofrequency devices has also provided an opportunity to improve dyschromia and photoaging, as well as fine lines and texture of the neck.[17–24] Although intense pulsed light and other monochromatic melanin-based wavelengths of light are very effective for brown and red "color correction," they have little effect on fine rhytides and wrinkles and the use of ablative fractional carbon dioxide lasers, and, to a lesser extent, ablative fractional and nonfractional erbium lasers can have the simultaneous benefit of decreasing the dyschromia and improving fine lines, rhytides, and laxity.[17–24] More recently, fractional radiofrequency devices, such as the Fractora (Invasix, Yokneam, Israel), have become available, which can provide variable depth and variable density needle-based tips for fractional ablative improvement of the dyschromia of the neck, as well as the textural improvements that can be equivalent to those achieved with carbon dioxide.[25] At the same time, the Fractora delivers a nonablative, non-necrotic tightening of the cervical region. The Fractora delivers radiofrequency energy and a positive charge along each of the pins in the needle array, resulting in an ablative crater and a zone of nonablative, but irreversible, thermal coagulation. Following the ablative injury, the radiofrequency (RF) energy then flows from the tip of the pin to the negative side electrode, creating a rich woven network of nonablative RF dermal heating, tightening, and remodeling (**Figs. 4–6**).[25]

Complications of the management of melanin and dyschromia of the neck include scars from overzealous laser and light-based settings, hypopigmentation from aggressive settings that result in a complete or near-complete clearance of melanocytes, as well as demarcation from treated and untreated areas.[6] Quite often, clinically, dyschromia occurs together with vascular discoloration, such as in Poikiloderma of Civatte, which is covered in the next section.

Vascular or hemoglobin-based cervical rejuvenation In addition to dyschromia and melanin-based lesions, it is quite common to get superficial vascular proliferation as a part of extrinsic photoaging or intrinsic genetic aging of

Fractora

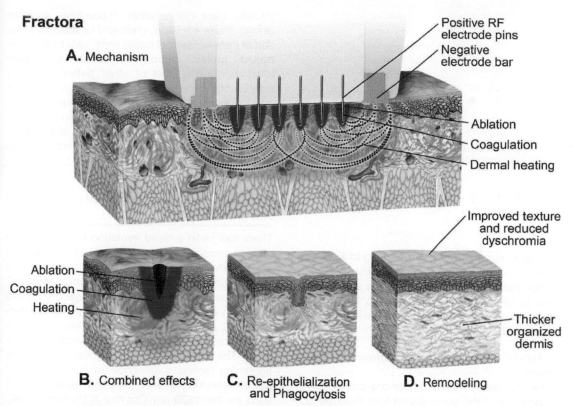

A. Mechanism

Positive RF electrode pins

Negative electrode bar

Ablation

Coagulation

Dermal heating

Improved texture and reduced dyschromia

Ablation
Coagulation
Heating

Thicker organized dermis

B. Combined effects

C. Re-epithelialization and Phagocytosis

D. Remodeling

Fig. 4. Fractora fractional radiofrequency resurfacing (*A*) showing the ablative crater and zone of non-ablative irreversible coagulation (*B*), re-epithelialization (*C*) and remodeling (*D*).

the neck. The vascular proliferation derived from photoaging responds very nicely to the intense pulsed light with the same cutoff filter spectrum mentioned in the dyschromia section.[11,14,15] Occasionally, deep dermal and subdermal, proliferative vascular lesions occur in the neck and monochromatic long-pulse or variable pulsed wavelengths, such as long-pulsed neodymium-YAG or short-pulse and long-pulse, pulsed dye lasers are required.[12] The combination of reticulated hyperpigmentation and vascular proliferation in the upper papillary and mid-dermis condition, called "Poikiloderma of Civatte," is more common in the lateral part of the neck than centrally. This "red neck syndrome" is often treated effectively with intense pulsed light, and peer-reviewed studies showing the successful use of a pulsed dye laser for this condition have been reported.[11–15] One of the complications of the treatment of vascular proliferation in the cervical region with monochromatic high-fluence, short-pulse duration lasers is only variable clearance of the

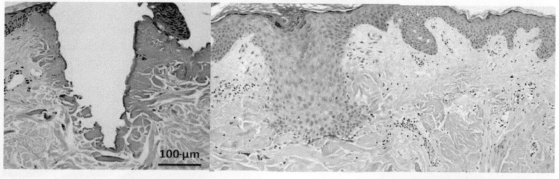

100 μm

Zone of Ablation and Coagulation

Re-Epithelialization   Re-Modeling

Fig. 5. High power histology showing fractora fractional RF ablative injury, with re-epithelialization and remodeling.

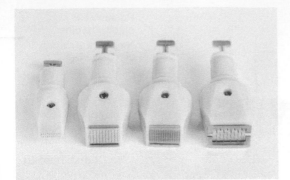

Fig. 6. The family of variable length and variable density Fractora tips.

reticulated hypopigmentation, leading to a partially white, "spotted leopard" look to the skin.[11–15] Intense pulsed light used gently over several sessions is often the best modality to blend most evenly the vascular as well as the melanin discoloration in the neck.

Epidermal and dermal nonchromophore-based lesions

There are many nonchromophore-based aging pathologies of the cervical skin that must be addressed to achieve the optimal outcome for

youthful neck rejuvenation. Procedures such as simple shave excision, chemical or thermal ablation of intra-epidermal papillomas, skin tags, compound moles, seborrheic keratosis, actinic keratosis, and a host of other pathologies can significantly improve the appearance of the neck (see **Fig. 6**). Superficial and deep dermal-epidermal rhytides can now be treated "off face" safely and effectively with fractional ablative lasers, CO2, Erbium, and fractional radiofrequency ablative systems (**Fig. 7**).[22–25]

Dermal and Subdermal Tightening Devices and Technologies

There has been a rapid evolution in our ability to provide moderate, nonexcisional skin tightening and wrinkle-reduction therapy with transepidermal energy devices. These new "energy-assisted" nonexcisional skin tightening procedures have become very important drivers of consumer interest, so it is critical that the aesthetic physician have a nonsurgical approach to cervical skin tightening. The first generation of the noninvasive skin-tightening technologies involved nonfractionated longer wavelength near infra-red laser devices, such as the 1320-nm Cooltouch (Roseville, CA), the 1440-nm Smoothbeam (Syneron Candela,

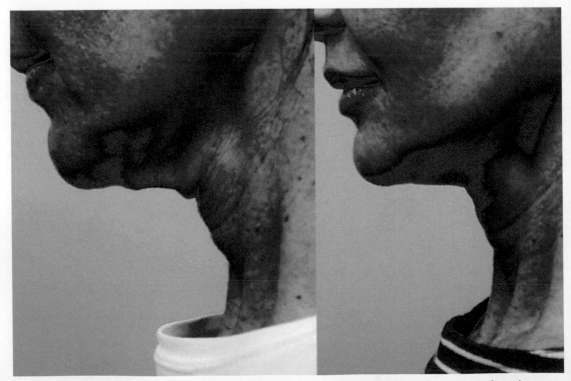

Fig. 7. Cervical rejuvenation with combined sub-dermal heating with Facetite for tightening, IPL for color correction, fractional RF ablative resurfacing for texture and CO2 shave excision of raised dermal and epidermal lesions.

Yokneam, Israel), the long-pulsed Nd:YAG, and the 1320 to 1440 nm synchronously pulsed Affirm MPX (Cynosure, Westford, MA).[26,27] The launch of externally applied RF devices provides the aesthetic physician with one of the most efficient "bulk heaters" of the dermis.[26–29]

Monopolar, stamping RF is typified by Thermage (Solta Medical, Hayward, CA), a very successful device with modest to good skin-tightening effects, proven in large multicentered trials.[28–35] Monopolar thermage protocols for treatment of the neck often includes 2 to 3 passes and 2 to 3 treatment sessions separated by several weeks. Combined optical-bipolar RF devices emerged, such as the Refirm and Polaris (Syneron), showing noticeable improvements using multiple-pass, multiple-session treatment protocols.[30–32] These mono-polar and bipolar RF or optical-RF combination devices, are "stamping" or "static" in nature and often suffer from inadequate dermal stimulation by a combination of very high peak dermal energy (and hence stimulation) but a very short pulse duration, exposing dermal tissue to a relatively short thermal stimulation that would be required for the production of new collagen, elastin, and ground substances. These stamping devices generally deploy protocols with multiple passes and multiple treatments to overcome the ultrashort pulse duration but high temperature model of collagen production stimulation.

More recently, a whole class of transepidermal RF heating devices have emerged that are not short-pulse duration "static" or stamping in nature, but rather, are continuous wave RF systems that are constantly moved along the surface of the skin along a thin layer of ultrasound or some interface gel. The advantage of these "moving" or "dynamic" RF systems is the ability to heat this tissue to a lower temperature but for a much longer period than pulsed mode stamping technologies and, depending on the "moving" device, the therapeutic thermal end point, usually 42°C to 43°C can be maintained, for a very long time. Some of the early "moving RF systems" include the Accent (Alma lasers, Buffalo Grove, IL), Tripolar (Polagen), the diamond polar and Octapolar (Venus Freeze [Venus Concept, Toronto, Canada]), the Excelis (BLT Industries Inc, Framingham, MA), and the 14 and 36 moving bipolar thermally controlled and modulated RF device, called the FORMA (Invasix).[35–44] The FORMA is a very high tech, thermally modulated enhanced moving RF heating device that has built within the hand piece sensors that measure high and low dermal impedance, epidermal temperature, and electrode contact 10 times every millisecond, and automatically adjusts RF energy depending on the sensory feedback. The FORMA will automatically cut the RF energy off when the therapeutic skin temperature is reached, the impedance drops too quickly (temperature is rising too quickly), or the electrodes lose contact with the epidermal surface.[43,44] Once the epidermis cools to 0.1°C below the target temperature, the RF energy is turned on again and heating resumes. The FORMA can read, modulate, and automate the high and low temperature extremes, keeping the skin at a very uniform and consistent thermal end point, usually 42° to 43° for prolonged periods of time by this process of thermal modulation and eliminating the "hot spots" that can cause patient discomfort and burns.[43,44] This thermomodulation process is called ACE, or *acquire, control, and extend*. The FORMA acquires the dermal-epidermal impedance, contact, and temperature information and will modulate the RF on and off, allowing the patient to experience a long, uniform, and comfortable period at the thermal end point (**Fig. 8**). As the thermal control is so exquisite, the patient rarely feels a thermal "hot spot" above 42° to 43° and the device burns can be greatly minimized and diminished. Clinical and histologic studies using ACE RF devices have shown good contraction and 14% more new collagen, and 35% collagen synthesis up-regulation.[44]

Over the past few years, fractional deep dermal ablative devices have been released and commercialized that can result in significant cervical skin rejuvenation. Ulthera, or fractional HIFU, uses high-frequency focused ultrasound to create ultrasound-induced fractional thermal ablative zones in the deep dermis and, in some areas, the superficial aponeurotic system. Results can be excellent, but occasionally painful and inconsistent.[45,46] The HIFU can be combined with IPL or other fractional ablative devices at the same session. Deep RF ablative needle devices are also commercially available, the ePrime (Syneron, Yokenim, Israel) uses an array of 6 bipolar, long silicon-coated RF-emitting needles inserted under local anesthesia to create deep microthermal ablative RF zones that result in remodeling and tightening, while sparing the epidermis. The Fractora family of applicators are available in different lengths and densities, with or without proximal silicone coating (**Fig. 9**). The 3000-μm pin tip (silicon coated or uncoated), alone or in combination with other more superficial Fractora high-density tips, can provide both ablative and nonablative tightening in the deep reticular and superficial papillary dermis. There is also a fractional RF resurfacing Fractora tip with 3000-μm pins that are coated with silicone proximally, to eliminate superficial

FORMA

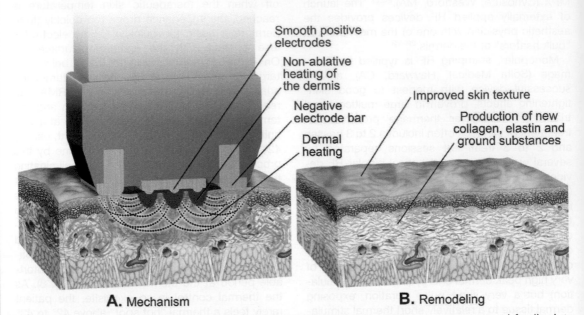

A. Mechanism

B. Remodeling

Fig. 8. The FORMA dynamic, non-ablative RF heating of the dermis. The FORMA uses sensors and feedback to continuously modulate the RF delivery dependent upon the measured epidermal temperature, high and low dermal impedance and contact sensing. The non-ablative heating, over a series of treatments results in 35% up-regulation of collagen synthesis and 14% more dermal collagen.

thermal stimulation and the epidermal risk of post-inflammatory hyperpigmentation, while delivering a selective deep dermal texture enhancement and skin-tightening effect (see **Fig. 9**; **Figs. 10** and **11**).

The 24-pin, 3000-µm silicon-coated tip, also called the Fractora Lift tip, is one of the more profound tightening fractional RF applications. The proximal 2000-µm silicone coating facilitates a selective deep dermal RF thermal ablation and nonablative coagulation (see **Fig. 10**). The 24-pin configuration and silicone coating offer a new generation of *bifractional stimulation*, horizontal and vertical fractionation. RF, being an efficient bulk heating energy, facilitates deep tissue remodeling without superficial thermal damage (see **Fig. 11**) The Fractora Lift tip can be used with various energies and multiple passes to result in tissue tightening of the brow, upper and lower lids, cheek, jawline, and neck, as well as deep line reduction and acne scar improvement. The silicone-coated tips can also be used off face. The Intracel, a fractional RF needle device, also uses silicone coating on its RF-emitting needles with variable energy and variable depth capability. The skin-tightening results of the these fractionated, vertical HIFU, or RF systems can be excellent to good, with, in general, one maintenance treatment every 3 to 6 months to "protect the

tightening" investment.[43–46] Thermally modulated nonablative skin-tightening applicators also can be used safely off the face and in combination with any other injectables and chromophore-based laser systems of fractional, ablative RF or laser systems.

The Subcutaneous Cervical Layer

Preplatysmal fat

Excessive preplatysmal fat will often compromise a youthful, acute cervicomental angle. There have been a myriad of ways developed over the past 30 years to address submental adiposity in a minimally invasive fashion. Suction-assisted lipoplasty (SAL), has been deployed for 3 decades to remove subcutaneous, preplatysmal fat and, hence, improve an oblique cervicomental angle and create a more youthful acute cervicomental angle.[47–51] SAL is still an excellent technique, particularly in those patients who have good skin tone and elasticity. SAL cannulas range from small, blunt, Mercedes-tipped cannulas, with vented ports, to flat spatula cannulas for separating the subdermal space from the preplatysmal subcutaneous tissue. Evidence exists that subdermal stimulation of the submental skin will likely improve skin contraction, but documented

Superficial, mid, and deep dermal, low and high density Fractora tips

A. Deep dermal, low density effects using the 3,000 micron, 24 pin array tip

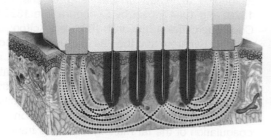

B. Mid dermal, high density effects using the 600 micron, 60 pin array tip

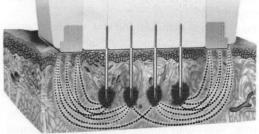

C. Mid dermal, high density effects using the 600 micron, 126 pin array tip

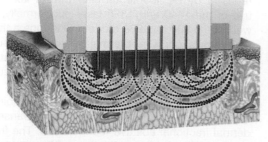

D. Superficial mechanical fractional injury and deep, low density fractional RF injury, using the silicone coated 3,000 micron, 24 pin tip

Fig. 9. The family of Fractora RF fractional resurfacing tip including the deep resurfacing 3000 micron tip (*A*), the mid-dermal low density 60 pin (*B*) and high density 126 pin (*C*) and the surface sparing bifractional silicone coated, 24 pin, 3000 micron Tip (*D*).

post-SAL retraction has generally ranged between 6% and 10% at 1 year postoperatively.[51–53]

To minimize ecchymosis and bruising, the introduction of ultrasound-assisted lipoplasty (UAL) in the 1990s brought a new option to the minimally invasive management of cervicomental contouring. Ultrasonic cavitation (streaming of fat cells) minimizes trauma to the subcutaneous vascular network, minimizing bruising, swelling,

and pain and optimizing a speedy postoperative recovery.[54–56] There are numerous articles that support the gentle nature of a UAL, and the Vaser from Sound Surgical (Solta Medical, Hayward, CA) is one the world's leading companies in this space. The incisional approach for UAL, like SAL is traditionally a submental stab incision, although for excess subcutaneous preplatysmal lateral adiposity, sublobular stab incision

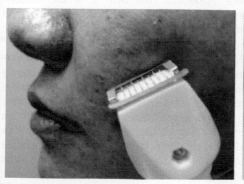

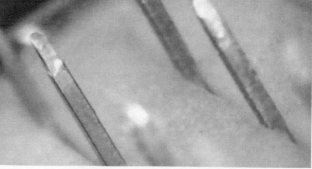

Fig. 10. The Fractora 24-pin, 3000 micron silicon-coated tip for deep dermal tightening with epidermal-dermal thermal sparing.

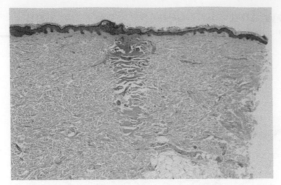

Fig. 11. High power histology showing the Fractora silicon-coated needle tissue effect with a non-ablative penetrating trauma superficially and a deep dermal thermal fractional injury with a superficial thermal sparing effect.

approaches have also been described and can be deployed.[54–56]

The challenge with SAL and UAL comes when a patient has some submental adiposity combined with skin laxity, decreased elasticity, and diminished elastic recoil. Patients with a large, modest, or even minor amount of fat, with poor skin tone, generally do not respond optimally to SAL or UAL, as the contraction is only a moderate 6% to 10%, even with strong, superficial, subdermal stimulation.[51–53] Many surgeons stand by their conviction and ability to stimulate the subdermal space with a nonthermal cannula achieving anecdotal reports of significant tightening; however, the experimental evidence of demonstrable skin contraction, with nonthermal superficial subdermal techniques, usually is reported to be in the 6% to 10% contraction range, when measured over 6 to 12 months.[50–52]

Increasingly, evidence-based medicine has shown that thermal techniques, both in the subcutaneous layer and in the subdermal layer, will lead to enhanced contraction well over and above those achieved with nonthermal, SAL and even UAL techniques.[52,53,57,58] One of the most popular and common options for submental, subdermal, and subcutaneous contouring is laser-assisted lipolysis (LAL).[52,53,57] Smartlipo, by Cynosure, is the world leader in this subdermal laser thermal stimulation market and there are published studies that show that raising the subdermal temperature to 50°C to 55°C, while keeping the epidermal temperatures under 40°C to 45°C, will achieve a 17% area soft tissue skin contraction over 3 to 6 months.[52,53] In addition, subdermal laser heating, to thermal end points, will result in increased dermal thickening of up to 25%, resulting from neo-collagenesis, as well as increased elasticity in the skin of 24%.[52]

The Smartlipo product, as well as other light laser lipolysis systems by other companies (SlimLipo by Palomar [Cynosure, Westford, MA], CoolLipo by CoolTouch [Roseville, CA], ProLipo by Sciton [Palo Alto, CA], and LipoLite by Syneron) all deploy a myriad of wavelengths: the 1440, 1320, and 1064 triplex by Cynosure; the 1320 by CoolTouch; the 1320 and 1064 by Sciton; the 1064 by Syneron; and the 924 and 967-nm diodes by Palomar. The various wavelengths in LAL are attracted to the water in the interstitial fluid created by the tumescent anesthetic technique and secondary cavitation of the tumescent fluid results in the thermal and non-thermal destruction and coagulation of the fat making for a less traumatic aspirate with decreased ecchymosis compared with SAL.[52,53] However, the principal goal of LAL is to induce the enhanced area contraction required by cervicomental skin that is lax. The use of the 1440 and 1320 laser subdermally, as well as the 927 and 968 diode, will induce a thermal stimulation. This thermal stimulation results in a deep reticular dermal collagen denaturization and the neo-collagenesis of the deep reticular layer and enhanced contraction.[52,53]

The use of subdermal LAL can be combined simultaneously and synchronously with transepidermal fractional ablative technologies. The fractional ablative lasers or fractional RF resurfacing devices can be deployed at relatively conservative energy levels synchronously with subdermal thermal techniques to induce a transepidermal fractional rejuvenation and tightening of the cervical soft tissue following the subdermal laser stimulation and aspiration. The fractional ablative lasers can be used alone for cervical texture and dyschromia therapy or in combination with cervical subdermal thermal techniques.

One of the newest and more compelling minimally invasive soft tissue tightening techniques of the neck is subcutaneous and subdermal RF-assisted lipocontouring (RFAL) (Invasix).[59–70] The Facetite applicator deploys a small, silicon-coated, 1.8-mm diameter, 13-cm long, solid RF-emitting probe with a bullet-shaped plastic tip to avoid subdermal "end hit" thermal injuries.[69] The FaceTite is a bipolar applicator with the internal and external electrodes and connected the by the hand piece. The RF current flows up from the internal to the external electrode, which glides along the epidermal surface in tandem with the RF-emitting internal electrode (**Figs. 12–14**). The FaceTite hand piece is connected to a console containing the RF card, electronics, and a central processing unit (CPU). The RF-emitting internal subdermal electrode coagulates subcutaneous fat in close proximity to the electrode in the

FaceTite effects on the dermis and epidermis

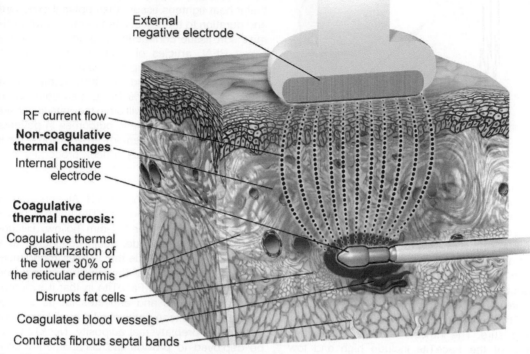

External negative electrode

RF current flow

Non-coagulative thermal changes

Internal positive electrode

Coagulative thermal necrosis:

Coagulative thermal denaturization of the lower 30% of the reticular dermis

Disrupts fat cells

Coagulates blood vessels

Contracts fibrous septal bands

Fig. 12. The FaceTite effect on the dermal and sub-dermal tissues coagulation of the immediate sub-dermal adipose tissue coagulation and then de-naturization.

Effects following use of the FaceTite

A. Non-ablative and coagulative changes

B. Remodeling

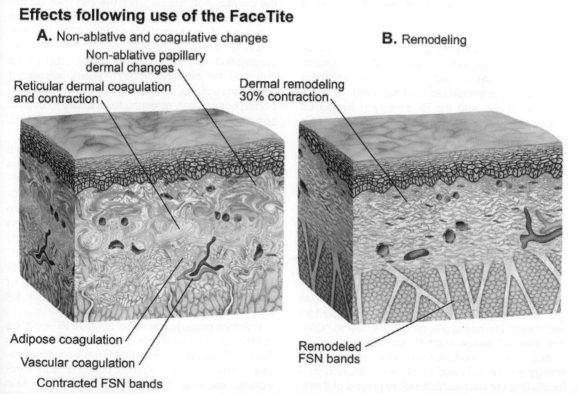

Non-ablative papillary dermal changes

Reticular dermal coagulation and contraction

Dermal remodeling 30% contraction

Adipose coagulation

Vascular coagulation

Contracted FSN bands

Remodeled FSN bands

Fig. 13. The FaceTite soft tissue effects with re-orientation of the immediate sub-dermal FSN and direct deep reticular dermal neo-collagensis re-modelling.

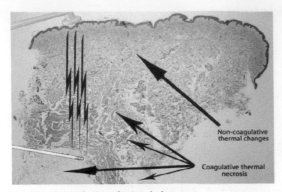

Non-coagulative thermal changes

Coagulative thermal necrosis

Fig. 14. Coagulative thermal changes.

superficial subdermal space and, as RF energy moves up to the external electrode, it dissipates and gently heats the papillary dermis. The coagulative heat of the subdermal fat results in a thermal denaturing of the reticular dermis, with preservation of the papillary dermis (see **Figs. 12–14**). The external electrode also contains a series of sensors that relay information to the console and CPU that can, in turn, respond by turning on or off the RF energy, modulating the thermal soft tissue exposure. The intricate and exquisite safety features of the FaceTite include high and low soft tissue impedance sensors, as well as epidermal contact sensors and an epidermal thermal sensor. This array of FaceTite safety sensors is able to detect rapidly rising dermal temperatures corresponding to rapidly dropping tissue impedance and are able to turn off the RF energy when these conditions approach empirically dangerous thermal levels. In addition, epidermal temperature is monitored and sampled 10 times per millisecond and the RF energy is turned off when the selected therapeutic end point is achieved. An epidermal temperature of 40° to 42° and a coagulative subdermal thermal exposure is the common end point. When the temperature of the epidermis decreases to 0.1°C below the target epidermal temperature, the RF energy is again turned on, much like an air-conditioning unit in the home and a constant subdermal temperature can be maintained.

This RFAL constantly modulated thermal system and internal impedance-monitoring process is called "ACE," whereby the RF device "*Acquires*" through sensors important information, such as low and high soft tissue impedance and contact and thermal temperature, allows the user to "*Control*" that soft tissue thermal exposure by an automated thermal modulation of the delivery of RF energy as the safe end points are met, and thus facilitating the user to "*Extend*" exposure of therapeutic soft tissue temperatures (hence, ACE, or Acquire-Control-Extend).

The safe, prolonged exposure of the subdermal tissue to heat, is predicated on the assumption that if heat tightens tissue, then optimal exposure and duration to therapeutic temperatures will optimize soft tissue contraction and tightening. Published RFAL articles on soft tissue contraction generally have shown up to a 25% area contraction at 6 months and 35–40% achieved at 1 year.[59–70] The 35–40% RFAL area contraction achieved at 12 months will often facilitate successful treatment and aesthetic outcomes in patients who might otherwise require an excisional neck procedure to have a closed neck procedure with aesthetically pleasing soft tissue contraction (**Fig. 15**).[62,68]

Another useful cervicomental RFAL applicator is called the NeckTite. The NeckTite (Invasix, Yokinem, Israel) is a larger 2.4-mm hollow, silicon-coated internal electrode, again connected to a similar external electrode that senses impedance, contact, and epidermal thermal monitoring. The NeckTite differs from FaceTite in that it synchronously coagulates and aspirates fat as well as heats, and for those patients who have large subcutaneous, preplatysmal adiposity, NeckTite can be deployed to provide the cervicomental contouring with reduction of adipose tissue (see **Fig. 15**). Depending on the laxity and elasticity of the cervical soft tissue, NeckTite can then be followed by a subdermal FaceTite applicator for enhanced dermal contraction (see **Fig. 15**). The NeckTite and its thermal stimulation relies on contraction of the adipose FSN (fibroseptal network) for contraction and, again, significant area contractions of 25% to 40% have been reported over 1 year, attesting to its ability to control soft tissue laxity more effectively than SAL or UAL (**Fig. 16**).[59–70]

Synchronous deployment of fractional ablative laser techniques on the epidermal-dermal surface immediately following subcutaneous and subdermal RFAL thermal stimulation will also induce additive contraction and textural and chromophore improvements. Alternatively, variable depth and density ablative fractional RF resurfacing therapy can be performed on the same session as subdermal RF (FaceTite) or laser thermal stimulation for an inside-outside dermal stimulation, with or without NeckTite stimulation of the deeper fat and FSN (**Fig. 17**).

Fractora deploys fractional ablative RF-emitting needles of various depths and densities that emit a fractional ablative energy that flows from the ablative craters to the negative charged side electrodes, creating a synchronous ablative skin injury and then a nonablative RF tightening as the RF current flows from the tip of the needle and

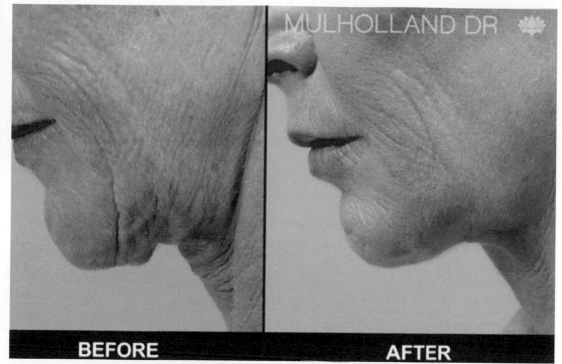

Fig. 15. Cervicomental contouring and enhancement with sub-dermal heating with FaceTite, submental fat reduction with Necktite and fractional ablative treatment with Fractora resurfacing.

NeckTite effects on the FSN and subdermal space

A. NeckTite mechanism   **B.** Effects immediately after use of NeckTite   **C.** Remodeling after NeckTite

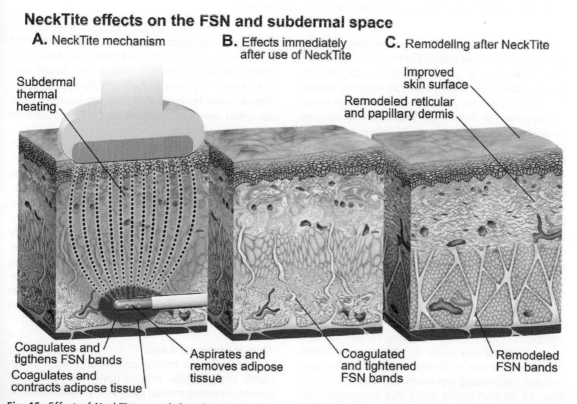

Fig. 16. Effect of NeckTite on subdermis.

Combining NeckTite, FaceTite, and Fractora

A. NeckTite   **B.** FaceTite   **C.** Fractora 3,000 micron, 24 pin tip   **D.** Fractora 600 micron, 60 pin tip

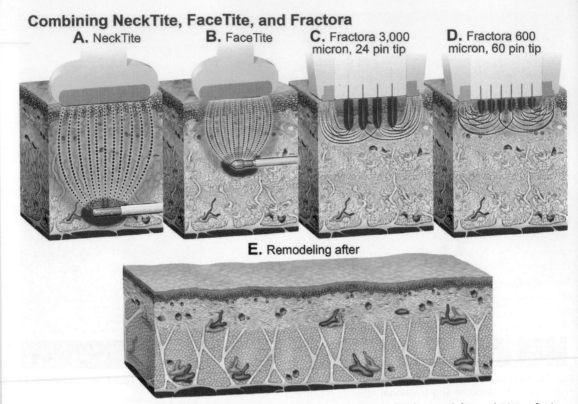

E. Remodeling after

Fig. 17. The combination of internal RFAL applicators for the reduction of submental fat and FSN soft tissue contraction, using NeckTite (*A*), sub-dermal skin tightening using FaceTite (*B*), Deep (*C*) and superfical ablative fractional RF resurfacing and non-ablative tightening with Fractora.

the base of the ablation through the deeper papillary and reticular dermis to the negative-side electrodes (see **Fig. 8**). Unlike fractional CO2, erbium, fractional RF resurfacing with this Fractora device can induce both an ablative rejuvenation of cervical dyschromia, fine lines, and rhytides, as well as nonablative deeper dermal cervical tightening. Simultaneous combination therapy, subdermal laser, or RF and transepidermal laser or RF, will often optimize the cervical rejuvenative therapeutic effect. The Fractora or other fractional ablative laser devices can be combined with IPL, laser, and other chromophore light-based systems together on the same visit with the FaceTite and/or NeckTite subdermal RFAL or subdermal laser to result in a multilayer cervical combination therapy that can optimize overall soft tissue color, texture, and contraction control.

There have been peer-reviewed studies reviewing the deployment of direct intra-adipose lipolytic injections in the submental space. These injections deploy substances such as phosphatidylcholine and deoxycholate to chemically damage the adipocytes, improving contour.[71–73] Modest reductions of fat can occur using this technique, but, like SAL or UAL skin contraction, would be limited

and color correction and texture improvement would necessitate the addition of light and energy-based systems.[73] There are newer adipose injection products being deployed for direct intra-adipose lipolysis that may hold some promise when used in combination with subdermal tightening techniques.

Platysma and cervical muscular layer

Deep to the subcutaneous adipose tissue is the platysma muscle. The platysma muscle is a thin straplike muscle that runs from the clavicle to the dermis of the mandible. It may or may not possess a medial decussation and, when taut, can create an enhanced and youthful cervicomental angle; but when lax, often creates visible and aging medial platysmal bands or cords and lateral platysmal bands. The anterior-posterior contraction of the platysmal muscles will also eventually lead to horizontal lines, or "necklace lines."

Medial platysma bands

Medial platysma bands can be divided into dynamic hypertrophic medial platysma bands and flaccid, atrophic medial platysma bands. Dynamic hypertrophic bands are usually more common in younger patients, and can compromise the cervicomental angle. Hypertrophic and dynamic medial platysma bands respond well to intramuscular injections of neuromodulators, such as botulinum toxin type A. This botulinum type A can include Botox, from Allergan (Irvine, CA), Dysport from Medicis/Valeant (Laval, Canada), and Xeomin from Merz (Frankfurt, Germany). Techniques for cervical injections include distraction and direct injection into the platysmal muscles, subcutaneous injections, or intradermal injections. The neuromodulator has a trophic capability to find its way to the presynaptic cleft of the motor axons in the platysmal muscle and provide a chemical denervation that prevents release of acetylcholine when one wants to activate the platysma bands. By chemically denervating the medial platysma bands, they will relax and in the dynamic hypertrophic patient, provide enhanced acuity of the cervicomental angle and reduced visibility of the aging appearance of the medial cords.[4,5] For the medial platysma bands, if the dynamic hypertrophic bands extend to the hyoid, doses of 15 units on either side can be deployed. If the bands extend below the hyoid to the level of the thyroid, or inferiorly to the sternal notch, another 15 to 30 units on either side of the platysma bands can be deployed. Care should be taken when injecting botulinum type A into platysma muscles that the injection is not performed too deeply or with copious amounts of neuromodulator, as cases of cervical dysphasia and swallowing difficulties have been reported, as well as difficulty lifting one's head due to sternocleidomastoid weakness.

Dynamic hypertrophic lateral platysma bands can also contribute to the aged appearance of the neck. The lateral platysma bands can act as a secondary depressors of the midface. Particularly when depressor angularis oris is blocked with botulinum toxin, lateral platysma hypertrophic patients will often overactivate the lateral platysma bands, creating a visually displeasing appearance to the neck, as well as causing a secondary depressed effect on the modiolus of the commissure and depressor effects on the midface. Direct Botulinum toxin A injection to the lateral platysma band, a procedure also called the "Nefertiti lift," has been advocated using 15 units used on either side.[4,5]

Anterior-posterior cervico and platysma flexion also create necklace lines. These can cause an aged appearance to the neck and multiple-site, low-dose intradermal or subcutaneous injections of botulinum type A, approximately 2 units every 2 to 6 cm along the entire necklace line, can provide a softening or rejuvenation of this region.[4,5]

The skin of the neck is very thin and the use of soft tissue fillers in cervical rejuvenation is somewhat limited, but for patients who have significant fine rhytides and horizontal lines, very dilute subdermal injections of particulate biostimulants such as Sculptra (polygalactic acid) can result in stimulation and a neo-collagenesis, with thickening of the dermis.[74,75] These techniques need to be performed with a very dilute solution (10:1 dilution) or fibroplastic nodules can result. Deploying very dilute hyaluronic acid gels in the subdermal space, as well as PRP (protein-rich-plasma) and other stem cell treatments, have also reported to provide reasonable rejuvenation of the neck. The neurotoxin and subdermal injectable biostimulants can, of course, be combined with transepidermal IPL on the neck to correct color and the fractional ablative techniques, RF or laser, for textural enhancement as discussed earlier in the article for combination therapy in neck rejuvenation. This kind of creative "combination therapy" can deliver outstanding soft tissue rejuvenation of the neck (see **Fig. 17**).

Laxity treatment of oblique cervicomental angle in the lax neck

Patients who have muscular laxity of the medial and lateral platysma muscle and obliquity of the cervicomental angle can often achieve nice aesthetic improvements with thread or suture suspension.[76–81] Two forms of suture suspension have been described in the literature, both of which have shown to provide nice results in selected patients:

1. Giampapa lift or suture suspension technique
2. Lateral suspension techniques or thread lifts

In the *Giampapa-lift or suture suspension technique*,[79] a small submental incision with elevation of flaps, allows visualization of the hyoid. Two interlinked polypropylene 4-0 or 3-0 nylon sutures are then passed through the hyoid periosteum. Following undermining of the lateral neck, with or without liposuction, again, the needle-based end of the polypropylene loop is then grabbed on both sides and passed using a very long clamp from the hyoid in the central neck to the retroauricular, mastoid space. Both ends of the now interlinked polypropylene suture are tightened and sutured to the mastoid and this creates an elevation of the hyoid, contouring the cervical soft tissue and enhancing the cervicomental angle.[79] In the properly selected patient, with a reasonable amount of subcutaneous adipose tissue, this can provide a pleasing and minimally invasive improvement. Of course, this suture suspension technique can be combined with any of the aforementioned subdermal and subcutaneous adipose-contouring techniques, subdermal-heating techniques, fractional ablative and light-based therapy, and neuromodulator techniques to enhance the results.

Lateral suspension techniques can be performed using various sutures that are either smooth or barbed or some type of resistance technology, such as cones, attached to the thread.[76–81] These lateral lifting techniques have generally been referred to as thread lifts and the most common techniques used in the neck incorporate fixation of the thread to the mastoid cervical fascia, although there were earlier suture-contouring technologies that did not incorporate solid fascial suture fixation.[78,79]

Simple polypropylene loops passed in the subdermal space and pulling the neck laterally and fixing the propylene to the cervical fascia can create modest improvements in the cervicomental angle. Barbed sutures or poly-l-galactic cones contained on a polypropylene backbone have been used and pass from lateral to medial to provide nice, significant early cervicomental contouring.[76,80,81] However, the long-term results of neck contouring using simple barbed or absorbable cone-based suture materials have generally resulted in a significant recurrence of cervicomental laxity, owing to extreme mobility of the neck and axial rotational movements. None of these lateral suture or device tension techniques deploy excision and the modest excess skin accumulates at the hair line and relaxes and remodels over time. Although short-term results can be favorable, there are very few reports of long-term cervical enhancements using these techniques, although further developments in the technology of suture and device suspension may improve the results from minimally invasive suspension cervicomental approaches.

Prominent digastric muscles

Occasionally, when large hypertrophic anterior bodies of the digastric are suspected of contributing to fullness of the immediate submental plane, in absence of significant fat, intramuscular botulinum toxin can reduce the fullness and improve the submental contour.[4,5]

Prominent submandibular glands

It is not uncommon for thin-necked patients to present with bulges in the submandibular space of the mandibular midbody. These bulges appear as displeasing shadows and are often a result of "low-hanging" submandibular glands.[3] The presence of prominent submandibular glands can be diagnosed through bimanual palpation (one finger on the floor of the mouth, one transcutaneous) and

feeling a smooth, soft glandular structure that often measures 4 to 5 cm in length and 1 to 3 cm in width. When submandibular glands are somewhat ptotic and enlarged, they can create an aged, shadowy appearance to the neck.

Botox has been deployed for the management of sialorrhea, both clinically and experimentally with reduction of saliva and histologically smaller glands.[82–84] The author has deployed a minimally invasive technique for managing enlarged, aesthetically displeasing submandibular glands by deploying botulinum toxin with direct injection into the submandibular gland, with 15 to 30 units of botulinum A per side. This glandular injection is most safely done with a bimanual technique (one finger in the floor of the patient's mouth, pushing on the submandibular gland, and the contralateral hand guiding the needle gently into the gland) or more recently with ultrasound guidance. I prefer to do this in 3 injection sites into each gland, with 5 to 10 units in each injection. Thirty units in each gland usually results in 9 to 12 months of resolution of the gland's visibility. Similar to axillary hyperhidrosis, the botulinum toxin acts presumptively on the acinar secretory apparatus, shrinking it significantly and minimizing the appearance of the submandibular gland for a prolonged period. Obviously, care and attention must be taken not to inject botulinum toxin into any other structure in the floor of the mouth (or your finger!) or some dysphasia or disarticulation can occur. The submandibular glands are functionally insignificant in the healthy patient, as the sublingual glands secrete most of the necessary salivary volume and prevent any xerostomia. However, in patients who have had oral carcinoma with oral radiation, the submandibular glands are best not injected, as xerostomia can result.

The aging neck remains one of the greatest challenges for the aesthetic physician. Minimally invasive, nonexcisional techniques to rejuvenate the midface and brow have delivered tremendous success for noninvasive head and neck surgeons over the past 5 to 10 years. Because of its structure, location, and, often, sun exposure, the cervical submental region has presented more challenges to the aesthetic physician in achieving consistent nonexcisional rejuvenation. Over the past few years, with the evolution of subdermal heating techniques and transepidermal fractional ablative techniques, chromophore-based and light-based systems, alone on in combination with subdermal stimulation and suspension techniques, the aesthetic physician now has many weapons and tools to better address the noninvasive and minimally invasive, nonexcisional treatments of the aging neck.

REFERENCES

1. US Census Bureau. Selected characteristics of baby boomers 42 to 60 years old in 2006. Washington: US Census Bureau; 2006.
2. Moretti, Michael. Skin tightening; softening demand in a weak economy. Aliso Viejo, CA: Medical Insight Inc; 2008.
3. Feldman J. Neck lift. St Louis (MI): Quality Medical Publishing Inc; 2006.
4. Carruthers A, Carruthers J. Cosmetic uses of botulinum exotoxin. Adv Dermatol 1997;12:325–47 Vancouver, Canada: Mosby-Year Book Inc.
5. Carruthers J, Carruthers A. The adjunctive usage of botulinum toxin. Dermatol Surg 1998;24:1244–7.
6. Schwartz RJ, Burns J, Rohrich RE, et al. Long term assessment of CO2 facial laser resurfacing: aesthetic results and complications. Plast Reconstr Surg 1999;103(2):593–601.
7. Bernstein LJ, Kauvar AN, Grossman MC, et al. The short and long-term side effects of carbon dioxide laser resurfacing. Dermatol Surg 1997;23(7):519–25.
8. Olsen EA, Katz HI, Levine N, et al. Tretinoin emollient cream for photodamaged skin: results of 48-week, multicenter, double-blind studies. J Am Acad Dermatol 1997;37:217–26.
9. Kang S, Leydon JJ, Lowe NJ, et al. Tazarotene cream for the treatment of facial photodamage. A multicenter, investigator-masked, randomized, vehicle-controlled, parallel comparison of 0.01%, 0.025%, 0.05% and 0.01% taxarotene creams with 0.05% tretinoin emollient cream applied once daily for 24 weeks. Arch Dermatol 2001;137:1597–604.
10. Anderson RR, Parish JA. Selective photothermolysis: a precise microsurgery by selective absorption of pulsed radiation. Science 1983;220(4596):524–7.
11. Sadick NS, Alexiades-Armenakas M, Bitter PH, et al. Enhanced full face skin rejuvenation using synchronous intense pulsed optical and conducted bipolar radiofrequency energy (ELOS): introducing selective radiophotothermolysis. J Drugs Dermatol 2005;4(2):181–6.
12. Zelickson BD, Kilmer SL, Bernstein E, et al. Pulsed dye laser for sun damaged skin. Lasers Surg Med 1999;25:229–36.
13. Weiss RA, Goldman MP, Weiss MA. Treatment of poikiloderma of civatte with an intense pulsed light source. Dermatol Surg 2000;26:213–8.
14. Bitter PH. Non-invasive rejuvenation of photodamaged skin using serial, full-face intense pulsed light treatments. Dermatol Surg 2000;26:9.
15. Bitter PH, Goldman MP. Non-ablative skin rejuvenation using intense pulsed light. Lasers Surg Med 2000;28(Suppl):12–6.
16. NegisThi K, Tezuka Y, Kushikata N, et al. Photorejuvenation for Asian skin by intense pulsed light. Dermatol Surg 2001;27(7):627–32.
17. Manstein D, Herron GS, Sink RK, et al. Fractional photothermolysis: a new concept for cutaneous remodeling using microscopic patterns of thermal injury. Lasers Surg Med 2006;34(5):426–38.
18. Geronemus RG. Fractional photothermolysis: current and future applications. Lasers Surg Med 2006;38(3):169–76.
19. Bass LS. Rejuvenation of the aging face using fraxel laser treatment. Aesthet Surg J 2005;25(3):307–9.
20. Daniel D, Bernstein LJ, Geronemus RG, et al. Successful treatment of acneiform scarring with CO2 ablative factional resurfacing. Lasers Surg Med 2008;40(6):381–6.
21. Chapas AM, Brightman L, Sukai S, et al. Successful treatment of acneiform scarring with CO2 fractional resurfacing. Lasers Surg Med 2008;40(6):382–6.
22. Gotkin RH, Sarnoff DS, Cannarozzo G, et al. Ablative skin resurfacing with a novel microablative CO2. J Drugs Dermatol 2009;8(2):138–44.
23. Rahman Z, Tanner H, Tournas J, et al. Ablative fractional resurfacing for the treatment of photodamage and aging. Lasers Surg Med 2007;39(s19):15.
24. Hruza G, Taub AF, Collier LS, et al. Skin rejuvenation and wrinkle reduction using a fractional radiofrequency system. J Drugs Dermatol 2009;8(3):259–65.
25. Mulholland RS, Ahn DH, Kreindel M, et al. Fractional radio-frequency resurfacing in Asian and Caucasian skin: a novel method for deep radiofrequency fractional skin resurfacing. J Chem Dermatol Sci Appl 2012;2:144–50.
26. Sadick NS. Update on non-ablative light therapy for rejuvenation: a review. Lasers Surg Med 2003;32:120–8.
27. Hardaway CA, Ross EV. Nonablative laser skin remodeling. Dermatol Clin 2002;20:97–111.
28. Fitzpatrick RE, Geronemus RG, Goldberg DJ, et al. Multicenter study of noninvasive radiofrequency for periorbital rejuvenation. Lasers Surg Med 2003;33:232–42, 14.
29. Dover JS, Zelickson BD. Results of a survey of 5,700 patient monopolar radiofrequency facial skin tightening treatments: assessment of a low-energy multiple-pass technique leading to a clinical end point algorithm. Dermatol Surg 2007;33:900–7.
30. Sadick NS, Trelles MA. Nonablative wrinkle treatment of the face and neck using a combined diode laser and radiofrequency technology. Dermatol Surg 2005;31:1695–9.
31. Sadick NS. Combination radiofrequency and light energies: electro-optical synergy technology in esthetic medicine. Dermatol Surg 2005;31:1211–7.

32. Sadick HS, Sorhaindo L. The radiofrequency frontier: a review of radiofrequency and combined radio-frequency pulsed-light technology in aesthetic medicine. Facial Plast Surg 2005;21: 131–8.

33. Friedman DJ, Gilead LT. The use of a hybrid radiofrequency device for the treatment of rhytides and lax skin. Dermatol Surg 2007;33:543–51.

34. Kist D, Burns AJ, Sanner R, et al. Ultrastructural evaluation of multiple pass low energy versus single pass high energy radiofrequency treatment. Lasers Surg Med 2006;38:150–4.

35. Mulholland RS. Radiofrequency energy for noninvasive and minimally invasive skin tightening. Clin Plast Surg 2011;38(3):437–48.

36. Emilia del Pino M, Rosado RH, Azuela A, et al. Effect of controlled volumetric tissue heating with radiofrequency on cellulite and the subcutaneous tissue of the buttock and thighs. J Drugs Dermatol 2006;5(8):714–22.

37. Mlosek RK, Wozniak W, Malinowska S, et al. The effectiveness of anticellulite treatment using tripolar radiofrequency monitored by classic and high frequency ultrasound. J Eur Acad Dermatol Venereol 2012;26(6):696–703.

38. Kaplan H, Gat A. Clinical and histopathological results following tripolar radiofrequency skin treatments. J Cosmet Laser Ther 2009;11(2):78–84.

39. Harth Y, Lischinsky D. A novel method of real-time skin impedance measurements during radiofrequency skin tightening treatments. J Cosmet Dermatol 2011;10(1):24–9.

40. Lee YB, Eun YS, Lee JH, et al. Effects of multi-polar radiofrequency and pulsed electromagnetic field treatment in Koreans: case series and survey study. J Dermatolog Treat 2012. http://dx.doi.org/10.3109/09546634.2012.714454.

41. Taub AF, Tucker RD, Palange A. Facial tightening with an advanced 4-MHz monopolar radiofrequency device. J Drugs Dermatol 2012;11(11): 1288–94.

42. Stampar M. The pelleve procedure: an effective method of facial wrinkle reduction and skin tightening. Facial Plast Surg Clin North Am 2011; 19(2):335–45.

43. Mulholland RS. Skin tightening in Asian patients using a dynamically controlled and thermally modulated radiofrequency energy device with ACE technology. Presented IMCAS Asia. Hong Kong, October 4–6, 2012.

44. Mulholland RS. Skin tightening in skin type 1-4 patients using a thermally modulated, feedback controlled, non-ablative radiofrequency device. Presented at IMCAS. Paris, Jan 31–Feb 3, 2013.

45. Suh DH, Oh YJ, Lee SJ, et al. An intense-focused ultrasound tightening for the treatment of infraorbital laxity. J Cosmet Laser Ther 2012; 14(6):290–5.

46. Alam M, White LE, Martin N, et al. Ultrasound tightening of facial and neck skin; a rater-blinded prospective cohort study. J Am Acad Dermatol 2010; 62(2):262–9.

47. Illouz YG. Body contouring by lipolysis: a 5-year experience with over 3,000 cases. Plast Reconstr Surg 1983;72:591–7.

48. Gasperoni C, Salgarello M, Emiliozzi P, et al. Subdermal liposuction. Aesthetic Plast Surg 1990;14: 137–42.

49. Goddio AS. Skin retraction following suction lipectomy by treatment site: a study of 500 procedures in 458 selected subjects. Plast Reconstr Surg 1991;87:66–75.

50. Matarrasso A. Superficial suction lipectomy: something old, something new, something borrowed. Ann Plast Surg 1995;24:268–72.

51. Toledo LS. Syringe liposculpturing. Aesthetic Plast Surg 1992;16:287–98.

52. DiBernado BE. Randomized, blinded, split abdomen study evaluating skin shrinkage and skin tightening in laser-assisted liposuction versus liposuction control. Aesthet Surg J 2010;30(4): 593–602.

53. Sasaki GH. Quantification of human abdominal tissue tightening and contraction after component treatments with 1064 nm/1320 nm laser-assisted lipolysis: clinical implications. Aesthet Surg J 2010;30:239–45.

54. Rohrich RJ, Beran SJ, Kenkel JM, et al. Extending the role of liposuction in body contouring with ultrasound-assisted liposuction. Plast Reconstr Surg 1998;101:1090–102.

55. Zocchi ML. Ultrasonic liposculpturing. Aesthetic Plast Surg 1992;16:287–98.

56. Zocchi ML. Ultrasonic assisted lipoplasty: technical refinements and clinical evaluations. Clin Plast Surg 1996;23:575–98.

57. Goldman A. Submental Nd:YAG laser-assisted liposuction. Lasers Surg Med 2006;38:181–4.

58. Prado A, Andreades P, Danilla S, et al. A prospective, randomized, double-blind, controlled clinical trial comparing laser-assisted lipoplasty with suction-assisted lipoplasty. Plast Reconstr Surg 2006;118:1032–45.

59. Paul M, Mulholland RS. A new approach for adipose tissue treatment and body contouring using radiofrequency-assisted liposuction. Aesthetic Plast Surg 2009;33(5):687–94. http://dx.doi.org/10.1007/s00266-009-9342-z.

60. Blugerman G, Schavelzon D, Paul M. A safety and feasibility study of a novel radiofrequency-assisted liposuction technique. Plast Reconstr Surg 2010; 125:998–1006.

61. Mulholland RS. An in-depth examination of radiofrequency assisted liposuction (RFAL). J of Cosmetic Surg and Medicine 2009;4:14–8.

62. Paul M, Blugerman G, Kreindel M, et al. Three-dimensional radiofrequency tissue tightening: a proposed mechanism and applications for body contouring. Aesthetic Plast Surg 2010;35(1):87–95 published with open access.

63. Paul MD. Radiofrequency assisted liposuction comes of age: an emerging technology offers an exciting new vista in non-excisional body contouring. Plastic Surgery Practice 2009;2:18–9.

64. Duncan DI. Improving outcomes in upper arm liposuction: adding radiofrequency-assisted liposuction to induce skin contraction. Aesthet Surg J 2012;32(1):84–95.

65. Theodorou SJ, Paresi RJ, Chia CT. Radiofrequency-assisted liposuction device for body contouring: 97 patients under local anesthesia. Aesthetic Plast Surg 2012;36(4):767–79.

66. Blugerman G, Schalvezon D, Mulholland RS, et al. Gynecomastia treatment using radiofrequency-assisted liposuction (RFAL). Eur J Plast Surg 2012. http://dx.doi.org/10.1007/s00238-012-0772-5. Published Online.

67. Divaris M, Boisnic S, Branchet MC, et al. A clinical and histological study of radiofrequency-assisted liposuction (RFAL) mediated skin tightening and cellulite improvement. J Chem Dermatol Sci Appl 2011;1:36–42.

68. Duncan DI. Improving outcomes in abdominal liposuction; comparing skin contraction with radiofrequency assisted lipocontouring (RFAL) plus SAL to SAL alone. Presented IMCAS. Paris, Jan 6–9, 2011.

69. Ahn DH, Mulholland RS, Duncan DI, et al. Nonexcisional face and neck tightening using a novel subdermal radiofrequency thermo-coagulative device. J Chem Dermatol Sci Appl 2011;1:141–6.

70. Hurwitz D, Smith D. Treatment of overweight patients by radiofrequency-assisted liposuction (RFAL) for aesthetic reshaping and skin tightening. Aesthetic Plast Surg 2012;36(1):62–71. http://dx.doi.org/10.1007/s00266-011-9783-z Published online.

71. Duncan DI. The evolution of mesotherapy. Presented at the ASPS Breast and Body Contouring Symposium. Santa Fe (NM), Oct 4–6, 2012.

72. Duncan DI. Injection lipolysis update. Presented at IMCA Asia. Hong Kong, Oct 4–6, 2012.

73. Rotunda AM. Mesotherapy and phosphatidylcholine injections: historical clarification and review. Dermatol Surg 2006;32:465–80.

74. Lam S, Azizzadeh B, Graivier M. Injectable poly-l-lactic acid (sculptra): technical considerations in soft-tissue contouring. Plast Reconstr Surg 2006;118:55–66s.

75. Beer KR, Rendon MI. Use of sculptra in esthetic rejuvenation. Semin Cutan Med Surg 2006;25:127–31.

76. Mulholland RS, Paul MD. Lifting and wound closure with barbed sutures. Clin Plast Surg 2011;38:521–35.

77. Ruff G. Techniques and uses for absorbable barbed sutures. Aesthet Surg J 2006;26:620–8.

78. Lycka B, Bazan C, Poletti E, et al. The emerging technique of the antiptosis subdermal thread. Dermatol Surg 2004;30:241–7.

79. Giampapa VC, DiBernado BE. Neck re-contouring with suture suspension and liposuction. Aesthetic Plast Surg 1995;19:217–24.

80. Gamboa GM, Vasconez LO. Suture suspension technique for the midface and neck rejuvenation. Ann Plast Surg 2009;62:478–81.

81. Mulholland RS. Advances and updates in barbed suture composite face and necklifts. Presented at IMCAS. Paris, Jan 9–12, 2008.

82. Coskun BU, Savk H, Cicek ED, et al. Histopathological and radiological investigations of the influence of botulinum toxin on the submandibular gland of the rat. Eur Arch Otorhinolaryngol 2007;264(7):783–7.

83. Breheret R, Bizon A, Jeufroy C, et al. Ultrasound-guided botulinum toxin injections for the treatment of drooling. Eur Ann Otorhinolaryngol Head Neck Dis 2011;128(5):224–9.

84. Shetty S, Dawes P, Ruske D, et al. Botulinum toxin type-A (Botox-A) injections for treatment of sialorrhea in adults: a New Zealand study. N Z J med J 2006;119(1240):U2129.

Progressive Tunnelizations in Neck Face Lift Detachment

Dilson Luz, MD

KEYWORDS

• Neck face lift • Face lift detachment • Facial hematomas • Nerve injury • Facial tunnelization

KEY POINTS

- Bleeding and facial nerve lesions are the greatest obstacles to a safe postoperative recovery in patients who undergo face and neck lift surgery.
- Hematoma complications are directly proportionate to the volume of blood accumulated and the time elapsed between the hematoma formation and its drainage.
- Complications typically occur from simple ecchymosis to cutaneous necrosis caused by excessive cauterization or tension on the closure.
- The Tunnelization in the subcutaneous plane technique emphasizes great attention to the liberation of the ligaments of the mandible, preserving the vascularity and the innervation in the ligament area. This is also performed in the middle third of the face.
- Patients who undergo face and neck lifting with detachment through progressive 'tunnelizations' show better recovery than those who undergo conventional rhytidoplasty, since they suffer less skin, vascular and nerve trauma performing cutaneous detachment with few cauterizations.

 A video of the author performing the progressive tunnelization technique accompanies this article online at http://www.plasticsurgery.theclinics.com/

Editor Commentary: I met Dilson while teaching in Brazil and was fascinated by his enthusiasm for a technique that seemed interesting and useful. Basically Dilson designed a series of dilators to perform blunt tunneling of the neck and face which allowed repositioning of soft tissues without extensive undermining with the added benefit of reducing the risk of hematoma formation. By squeezing the vessels in the flap, there is virtually no bleeding, explained in his section on physiology, and when I added this to my routing necklift technique, I enjoyed infrequent accumulations of blood and seroma fluid in the neck. I also found this step valuable in decreasing the risk of skin loss in smokers as I did not detach the neck flap, leaving important fasciocutaneous perforators to nourish a flap whose circulation may be compromised.

INTRODUCTION

Face-lifting surgery is progressing through clinical research and documentation of results as well as sequelae, complications, and longevity (Video 1). The round-lifting technique described by Pitanguy and colleagues[1] and based on a directional study of the vector for the lifting of sagging skin, as well as the necessary skin incision, reflects the search for efficiency in facial surgery. The changes in incisions have shown vast progress, securely preventing the elevation of the sideburn with the peninsula technique idealized by Pontes.[2] Mitz and Peyronie[3] established the anatomic basis for the superficial musculoaponeurotic system (SMAS) treatment, additionally defining that the SMAS adherences to the parotid fascia form a fixed tissue

Brazilian Society of Plastic Surgery and International Society Aesthetic Plastic Surgery (ISAPS), Av Engenheiro Domingos Ferreira, 636, Sala 310, Boa Viagem, Recife, Pernambuco 51011-050, Brazil
E-mail address: dfluz@yahoo.com.br

Clin Plastic Surg 41 (2014) 33–41
http://dx.doi.org/10.1016/j.cps.2013.09.001
0094-1298/14/$ – see front matter © 2014 Elsevier Inc. All rights reserved.

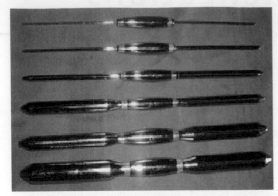

Fig. 1. Dilson Luz Vascular Dilation Wands used for skin detachment with progressive tunnelizations.

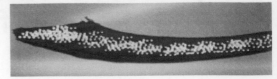

Fig. 3. Trapped blood clots in the extremities of the sectioned vessels.

and that anterior to the parotid the SMAS is mobile. Hakme[4] claims (and the author agrees) that the treatment of the SMAS (with imbrication or with SMASectomy) only maintains the results if the movable SMAS is sutured to a fixed base. There are instructions about how to avoid nerve lesions[5] and precise anatomic descriptions for interventions in the premasseteric space (Mendelson and colleagues[6]), collaborate in the prevention of complications. Vasconez and colleagues[7] defined the basis for video-endoscopic facial surgery, and Badin and colleagues[8] are credited with the surgery with vector modifications and wire traction. In addition, the critiques and evaluations of complications from the use of a barbed suture, mentioned by Paul,[9] reflect the masters' concerns in guiding the future generations with safety.

Despite so much research and technological innovations, the bleeding problems caused by surgery, as well as the attempts to minimize its complications, persist. The facial nerve lesions continue equally frequently, even in experienced hands and with the use of preventive procedures.

Based on the author's experience and on extensive bibliographic research, he ascertains that bleeding and facial nerve lesions are the greatest obstacles to a safe postoperative recovery in patients that undergo face- and neck-lift surgery.[10]

In order to have more dense and uniform skin flaps (because the subcutaneous vascular plexus is mostly responsible for skin irrigation[11]), reduce bleeding during surgery, avoid immediate or late postoperative hematoma formation, and minimize the risks of facial nerve lesions, the author would like to present his technique, which is a pioneering effort in face and neck lifting: detachment with progressive tunnelizations using the Dilson Luz Vascular Dilation Wands (Mad Colant, Jaboatão, Pernambuco) (**Fig. 1**). This technique can be applied in other surgeries,

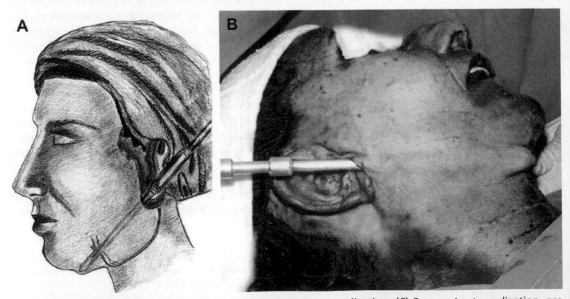

Fig. 2. (*A*) Liberation of mandible ligaments with progressive tunnelization. (*B*) Progressive tunnelization, prolonging detachment of middle third of face.

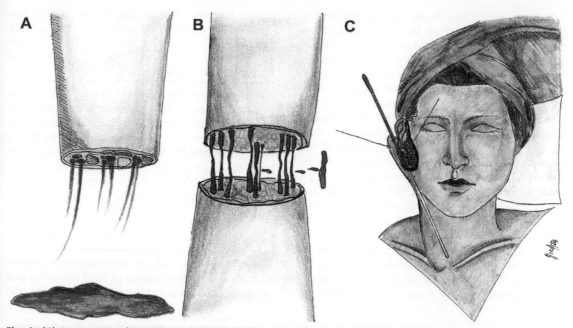

Fig. 4. (*A*) Amputation for pullout presents minimal blood loss. (*B*) Amputation via sharp object causes hemorrhage. (*C*) Concept of major bleeding applied to neck and face detachment.

such as lipo-abdominoplasty, prosthesis inclusion in calves and breasts, inclusions of expanders, breast reconstructive surgery, and glutoal muscle lifts.[12] This technique was used and reproduced with success.[13]

In surgeries performed through classic techniques, the manual drainage of the collected blood from the hemifaces already sutured are common, and cases of the removal of stitches to check the hemostasis at the end of the surgery are not rare. It is common knowledge among surgeons that the return of patients to surgical centers to check for hematomas happens with a certain frequency. These patients are not always exempt from complications, which are directly proportionate to the volume of blood accumulated and the time elapsed between the hematoma formation and its drainage. Usually, complications occur from a simple ecchymosis to cutaneous necrosis, accompanied or not with neurologic lesions caused by cauterization or section of nerves.[14]

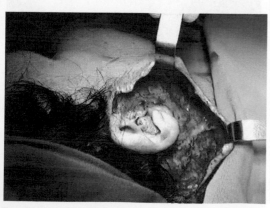

Fig. 5. More dense flaps result from infiltration with greater tumescence.

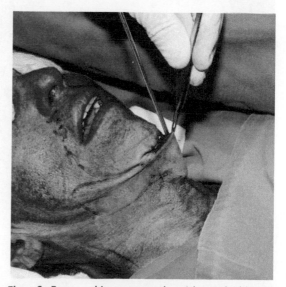

Fig. 6. Excess skin managed with rods/dilators, completing the progressive tunnelizations on the entire neck, until total cutaneous stretch.

In the author's technique, special attention is given to the ease of doing the detachment of the neck and of the middle third of the face (which is divided into superficial and profound), safely guiding the liberation of the zygomatic ligaments through the profound detachment supraperiostal tunnelized and progressive superficial detachment for the elevation of the malar fat pad. The author emphasizes the care for the liberation of the ligaments of the mandible, prolonging the detachment of the middle third superficial, tunnelizing progressively in the subcutaneous plane for these ligaments, observing the vascularization, the innervation, and the ligament area (**Figs. 2** and **3**) (becomes **Fig. 2**A, B), which was so well demonstrated by Furnas.[15]

In 2003, the author presented his technique for the first time.[16] In 2005, the author published his technique in *Aesthetic Plastic Surgery*[17]. In 2006, the author published it in an Brazilian Society of Plastic Surgery - Region São Paulo (SBCP) São Paulo book; in 2010, he edited his book on the technique.[18]

Technique Fundamentals

The physiology is explained by the vascular intima section that provokes the platelet migration to the injured area, following the immediate coagulation within the vascular extremities, because these were submitted to a progressive stretching with large dilators in its lights before the section, obtaining trapped clots in the extremities of the sectioned vessels, which block the blood flow (see **Fig. 3**).[19]

Physiology

The observation that, in emergencies, patients who underwent amputation of their hands by pull out presented minimum blood loss (**Fig. 4**A) and

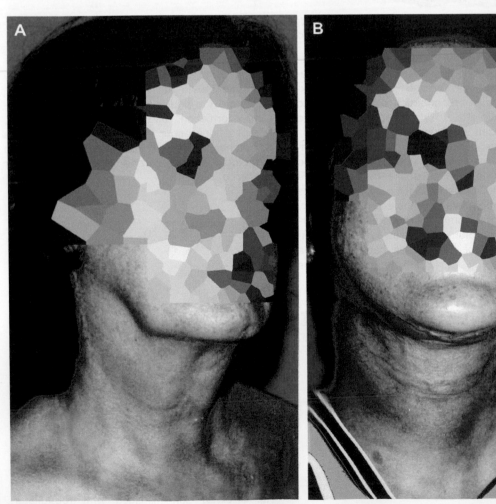

Fig. 7. Subcutaneous progressive tunnelizations performed on the lateral neck and extending to the clavicle region. (*A*) preoperative and (*B*) postoperative.

that patients who suffered identical amputation but caused by sharp objects suffered from severe anemia (see **Fig. 4**B) raised the question of how to prevent hemorrhaging during the detachment of the face. The author transferred this idea to perform the neck-face detachment (see **Fig. 4**C).

PATIENT SELECTION

Currently, the author thinks that his technique is indicated in all patients submitted to face- and neck-lifting surgery and especially in those who present with acute cervical flaccidity extended to the clavicle region and in those that present risks of blood pressure variation during surgery.

SURGERY DESCRIPTION
Preoperative Marking

The markings of face and neck lifting are initially done with patients seated in the hospital room, according to the surgery plan previously discussed and analyzed in the consultation room. These markings are supplemented in the surgical center.

Anesthesia

All of the patients underwent surgery while under local anesthesia with sedation and monitored by an anesthesiologist. Using fine cannulas (1.0–1.5 mm), the infiltrations were done with lidocaine 0.5% and adrenaline solution 1/200.000 (1/400.00 for tumescence) in a variable volume of 200 to 300 mL for the entire neck and the face. The infiltrations were started previously in the areas where surgery was to take place. In thin patients, there was a need for infiltration with greater tumescence to obtain more dense flaps (**Fig. 5**). It was also noticed that the cannulas' infiltrations reduce the amount of ecchymosis and prevent vascular penetration of the anesthetic, preventing blood pressure elevations and/or lesions of the facial nerve by needle trauma during surgery.

Neck Treatment

After blepharoplasty and eyelid elevation, when needed, the neck lift is initiated.

Cervical Liposuction

When necessary, cervical liposuction is done with 20-mL syringes and fine cannulas in the areas previously marked.

Incision and Detachment

With the cutaneous incision of 3 to 4 cm, parallel and below 2 to 3 mm from the submental fold,

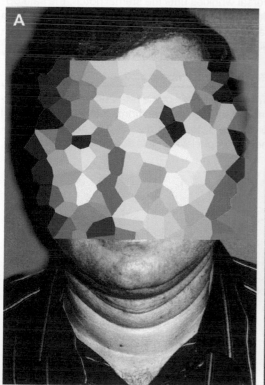
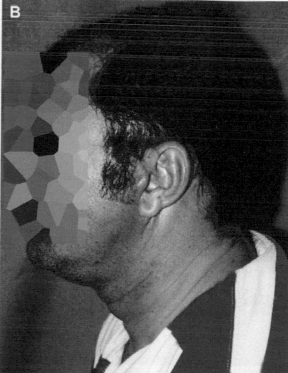

Fig. 8. Neck with acute flaccidity without fat to be aspirated, showing transversal wrinkles to the sternal notch. (*A*) preoperative and (*B*) postoperative.

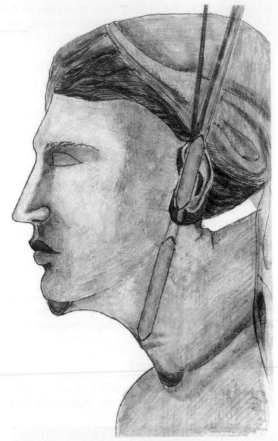

Fig. 9. Immediately below the retroauricular region, the subcutaneous detachment is initiated with progressive tunnelizations until it has continuity with detachments of the cervical portion.

the detachment is initiated with progressive tunnelizations of the medial portion and the rest of the neck, previously aspirated, when needed. The author returns to the medial portion with larger

rods/dilators until the platysmal bands are identified and performs the hemostasis immediately with few cauterizations.

After the plication, the author performs vertical ellipse and/or sections of the platysmal bands, with the excision of the subplatysmal fat and excessive bands, when necessary. When excess skin is present in the central region of the neck without cutaneous stretch (**Fig. 6**), this condition will be treated with rods/dilators, completing the progressive tunnelizations on the neck, until total cutaneous accommodation.

It was observed that the subcutaneous progressive tunnelizations can be done safely on the lateral neck and below, when necessary, extending to the clavicle region (**Fig. 7**). Doing so, it is possible to accommodate all the inferior cervical skin with small and medium rods/dilators. The larger rods/dilators are used to complete the lateral tunnelizations and the ones below the mandibular ramus, which will have continuity with tunnelizations in the middle third, avoiding the need for cauterization in the area where the rods/dilators are used (see **Fig. 5**). The procedure is completed with the suturing of the submental fold, through which a laminar drain is inserted.

In the case of a neck with acute flaccidity without fat to be aspirated, but showing transversal wrinkles until the sternal notch, the safe option for the procedure is to use rods/dilators to raise the cervical skin with progressive tunnelizations (**Fig. 8**).

Retroauricular Region

The glabrous skin of the retroauricular region is detached through the traditional method, with scalpel or scissors, to get a denser flap of skin for cutaneous prophylaxis in this area. Immediately below,

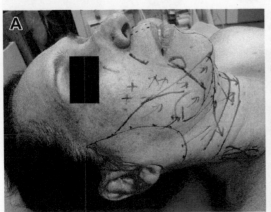
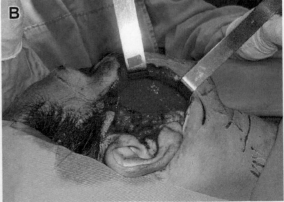

Fig. 10. (*A*) Detachment of middle third of face with tunnelization of the supra-SMAS through the classic preauricular incision or from short scar approach. (*B*) Return to the preauricular area marked for total detachment through insertion of larger rods/dilators to view the SMAS area for treatment.

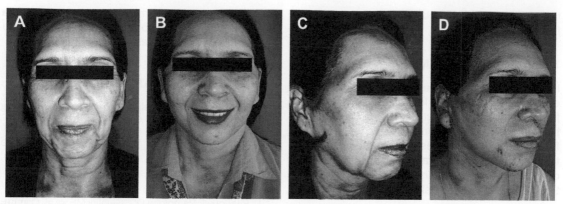

Fig. 11. Elevation of the middle third of face via trabeculars and sufficient tunnels after profound tunnelization supraperiosteal with small and medium rods/dilators, above the malar fat pad. (*A* and *C*) preoperative; (*B* and *D*) postoperative.

the subcutaneous detachment is initiated with progressive tunnelizations until it has continuity with the detachments of the cervical portion (**Fig. 9**).

To clarify how the applications of these progressive tunnelizations complete the neck lift, the surgery on the third middle of the face is described:

The detachment begins with the tunnelization of the supra-SMAS through the classic preauricular incision or from the short scar approach (**Fig. 10**A). The small rods/dilators penetrate the subcutaneous space forming tunnels, freeing above the masseteric ligaments' adherences and below the mandibular ligament in its cutaneous insertions. The tunnels below overtake the inferior labiomental sulcus and, with small and medium rods/dilators, will have continuity with the previously detached neck tunnels (see **Fig. 2**).

After these tunnelizations, the author returns to the preauricular area marked for total detachment, which is achieved by inserting larger rods/dilators to rupture the trabeculars and make it possible to view the SMAS area for treatment (see **Fig. 10**B).

The area described by Aston,[20] in Finger assisted malar elevation (FAME), will be profoundly tunnelized supraperiosteally with small and medium rods/dilators, above the malar fat pad, and the periosteal insertion of the zygomatic ligament, leaving trabeculars and only sufficient tunnels for

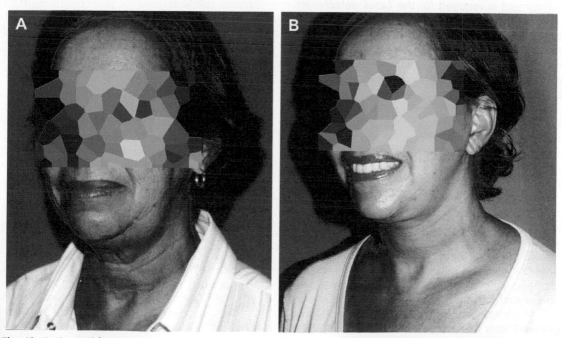

Fig. 12. Patient with ptosis of the submandibular gland treated with platysmal plication. (*A*) preoperative; (*B*) postoperative.

the necessary elevation of the middle third of the face (**Fig. 11**).

TREATMENT OF THE SMAS

In conclusion, the treatment of the SMAS is usually done with imbrication, fixing the movable SMAS to fixed points with nylon sutures 3.0 and maintaining the malar fat elevated and fixed to the temporal fascia[8] with nylon sutures 2.0. Hemostasis is obtained with few cauterizations; after the excision of extra skin, the author inserts laminar drains, sutures, and applies occlusive bandages.

DISCUSSION AND SUMMARY

Patients subjected to face and neck lifting with detachment through progressive tunnelization show better recovery than those subjected to conventional rhytidoplasty because they experience less trauma because of fewer cauterizations. Furthermore, patients show less vascular and nerve lesions because this technique leaves trabeculars that form tunnels resulting in less dead space. All of these factors result in less morbidity, enabling patients to return to regular activity sooner.

The learning curve is rapid, and the procedure using the rods/dilators is reproducible because the detachment is done in the same plane as the traditional way, except that there is no bleeding as is seen with the scalpel or scissors. A small adjustment is required for the facial detachment when using rods/dilators in a progressive manner, seeking to view the edge of the rods/dilators in all its subcutaneous extension, in the surface of the detachment with scissors, with exception to the malar region, where the tunnelizations are made in the profound surface.

The detachment with progressive tunnelizations applied to the neck becomes a unique process that is capable of safely treating the flaccidity of the inferior third, many times forming tunnels progressively until the clavicle region and largely eliminating cauterizations.

A total of 372 patients were subjected to this new technique since 1999; all of them were accompanied up until the present time with no irreversible cases of damage to the facial nerve. There were 2 cases of neuropraxias that lasted from 4 to 8 weeks; after the author began using tumescent infiltrations, they no longer appeared. There were no patients with cutaneous necrosis and/or formation of hematomas during the immediate or late postoperative phases. Patients with ptosis of the submandibular gland were treated with platysmal plication and were satisfied (**Fig. 12**). Other plastic surgeons have reaffirmed that the technique described is reproducible, and they have reached results as satisfactory as the author's.

SUPPLEMENTARY DATA

Supplementary data related to this article can be found online at http://dx.doi.org/10.1016/j.cps.2013.09.001.

REFERENCES

1. Pitanguy I, Pamplona DC, Giuntini ME, et al. Computational simulation of rhytidectomy by the "round-lifting" technique. Rev Bras Cir 1995;85:213–8.
2. Pontes R, editor. Universo da Ritidoplastia. Rio de Janeiro (Brazil): Revinter; 2011. p. 119–46.
3. Mitz V, Peyronie M. The superficial musculo-aponeurotic system (SMAS) in the parotid and cheek. Plast Reconstr Surg 1976;58:80–8.
4. Hakme F. SMAS-platisma nas ritidoplastias cérvico-faciais. Rev Bras Cir Plast 1982;72:105–10.
5. Dingman RO, Grabb WC. Surgical anatomy of the mandibular ramus of the facial nerve based on the dissection of 100 Facial halves. Plast Reconstr Surg 1962;29:266–72.
6. Mendelson BC, Freeman ME, Wu W, et al. Surgical anatomy of the lower face: the premasseter space, the jowl, and the labiomandibular fold. Aesthetic Plast Surg 2008;32:185–95.
7. Vasconez LO, Core GB, Gumboa-Bobadilla M, et al. Endoscopic techniques in coronal brow lifting. Plast Reconstr Surg 1994;94:788–93.
8. Badin AZ, Casagrande C, Roberts T, et al. Minimal invasive facial rejuvenation endolaser mid-face lift. Aesthetic Plast Surg 2001;25:447–53.
9. Paul MD. Complication of barbed sutures. Aesthetic Plast Surg 2008;32:149.
10. Cardoso de Castro C, Aboudib JH Jr. Complicações: cirurgia de rejuvenescimento facial. Rio de Janeiro (Brazil): Médica e Científica Ltda; 1998. p. 321–41.
11. Schaverien MV, Pessan JE, Rohrich RJ. Vascularized membranes determine the anatomical boundaries of the subcutaneous fat compartments. Plast Reconstr Surg 2009;123:695–700.
12. Luz D, editor. Técnica Dilson Luz–Tunelizações Progressivas: Princípios, Aplicações e Procedimentos Complementares. 1st edition. Rio de Janeiro (Brazil): Di Livros; 2010.
13. Luz DF, editor. Técnica Dilson Luz Tunelizaciones Progresivas, Principios, Aplicaciones y Procedimientos Complementarios. 2nd edition. Bogotá (Colombia): Impresion Medica; 2012.
14. Franco T, Ribeiro C. Ritidoplastias: cirurgia Estética. 1st edition. Rio de Janeiro (Brazil): Atheneu; 1991. p. 49–110.

15. Furnas DW. The retaining ligaments of the cheek. Plast Reconstr Surg 1989;83:11–6.

16. Luz DF. Técnica Dilson para o descolamento na cirurgia do Face-Liftig-Profilaxia de hematomas e lesões do nervo facial. Brasilia (Brazil): Jornada Centro Oeste C.P; 2003.

17. Luz DF, Wolfenson M, Figueiredo J, et al. Full-face undermining using progressive dilators. Aesthetic Plast Surg 2005;29:95–9.

18. Luz DF, editor. Técnica Dilson para o descolamento na cirurgia do Face-Lifting-Profilaxia de hematomas e lesões do nervo facial. São Paulo (Brazil): Robe Editorial; 2006. p. 115–24.

19. Weis HJ. Hole of platelets in blood physiology. Clin Cir Am N 1988;4:810–3.

20. Aston SJ, editor. The fame technique presented at the aging face symposium. New York: Waldorf Astoria; 1993.

Lore's Fascia a Strong Fixation Point for Neck Rejuvenation Procedures

Athanasios Athanasiou, MD, PhD[a],*,
Georgios Rempelos, MD[b]

KEYWORDS

- Neck rejuvenation • Procedures • Neck lift • Platysma muscle

KEY POINTS

- Lorre's fascia as anchor point provides strong support to the young hanging neck without the need for further subplatysmal dissection.
- An additional subplatysmal dissection and submental approach with liposuction and digastric manipulation addresses problems of heavier problematic necks.
- Facial contour is restored in a natural, long-lasting result.

 The authors present a brief video clip of their skin fixation in neck rejuvenation accompanies this article at http://www.interventional.theclinics.com/

Editor Commentary: Athanasias spent a six month aesthetic fellowship with me and frequently visited Bruce Connell as well. He shares his answers to my questions in a logical manner utilizing the strength of Lore's fascia and the mastoid fascia to anchor the SMAS/platysma flap. These fixed structures limit anterior and inferior flap migration after anchoring. He describes his approach to the various layers of submandibular fat as well as the indication for partial resection of the anterior belly of the digastrics muscles. His European patient population includes many smokers and his admonition to avoiding aggressive flap dissection is important to remember.

TECHNIQUE
Managing Aging Necks

The surgical necessity to individualize each patient's needs to one specific technique enabling the surgeon to offer a satisfactory result in all varieties of an aging neck is meaningless.[1–15] From our experience, there is no one-for-all technique to address every anatomic area found in existing or potential problems on the constantly shrinking neck cylinder. Skin flaccidity, supraplatysmal or subplatysmal excess fat, mandibular border definition, visible active or static platysma muscle bands, and submaxillary gland protrusion form

a certain reconstructive ladder that guides our surgical steps. Our neck lift procedure is a combined chain of these steps with a sense of priority. Our responses to the questions asked are as follows:

What incisions do you typically use in the thin neck and the heavy neck in both young and older patients?

Skin-incision length is roughly guided by the degree of skin laxity. Limited skin incisions (or short scar lifts) are best suited for young candidates with mild excess skin and more soft tissue loss

[a] Private Practice, Laodikis 33-35 Glyfada, Greece; [b] Private Practice, 64 L. Riankour street, 16B suite, Apollo tower, 11523 Ampelokipi, Athens, Greece
* Corresponding author.
E-mail address: tanasisa@yahoo.gr

Clin Plastic Surg 41 (2014) 43–49
http://dx.doi.org/10.1016/j.cps.2013.09.008
0094-1298/14/$ – see front matter © 2014 Elsevier Inc. All rights reserved

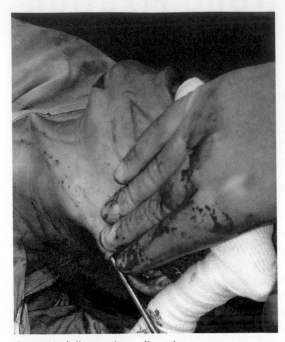

Fig. 1. Neck liposuction - dissection.

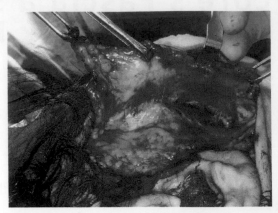

Fig. 3. Extended SMAS mobilization for neck rejuvenation.

A submental approach is being introduced in our surgical protocol when a pinch test indicates the presence of a substantial amount of subplatysmal fat that requires open cervical lipectomy. A 3- to 4-cm incision is then placed about 1 cm inferiorly to the submental crease to provide better healing conditions, an inconspicuous scar, and to avoid the double-chin deformity. If the neck skin is loose, then we extend the incision behind the earlobe, leaving a 3-mm cuff of skin below the junction to the cheek (**Figs. 2** and **3**). The incision is carried backward following the earlobe-postauricular skin junction and, at the level of the tragus (or sometimes 5 or 10 mm higher), is turned toward the hairline with a cutting angle parallel to the hair follicles, with a special effort to preserve them. Through this incision, we can remove large amounts of flaccid skin, avoid unpleasant folds, and respect the natural relaxing lines of the neck. In this way, we avoid the danger of creating a pulled look, which is a disfiguring disadvantage of various U-shaped incisions (**Fig. 4**).

of support. Usually the midface is not yet affected, so no high superficial muscular aponeurotic system technique or extended excision is required. Lateral surgical excision of SMAS or plication is enough to correct the descending face and neck. We think that using the mastoid and Lorre's fascia as anchor points provides strong support to the young hanging neck without the need for further subplatysmal dissection. If supraplatysmal fat is problematic, it can be suctioned using a flat cannula with a special effort not to skeletonize the submandibular area and, therefore, reveal an enlarged submandibular gland or a prominent anterior digastric belly (**Fig. 1**).

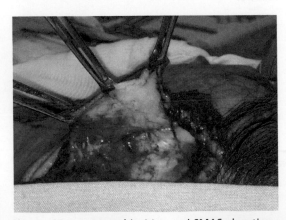

Fig. 2. Skin retrotragal incision and SMAS elevation.

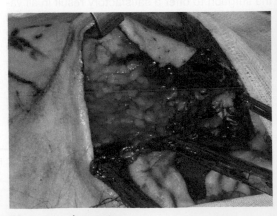

Fig. 4. Ancoring vectors.

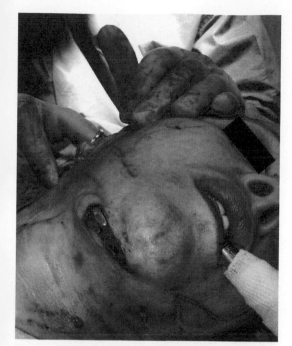

Fig. 5. Unification of surgical planes.

What is your approach to defatting the heavy neck? Which fatty layers do you resect (ie, subcutaneous, interplatysmal, subplatysmal fat)?

A limited superficial liposuction is performed in the submental area before our face procedures. The purpose is not a precise preplatysmal fat removal rather than an atraumatic dissection on the supraplatysmal plane of the neck. The skin flap is raised using the 4-handed technique under direct vision aided by transillumination, and the dissection proceeds to the avascular plane about 1 cm medial to the anterior border of the sterno-cleidomastoid muscle. Then the surgical plane is divided, and the superficial part is connected to the previous liposuction plane where fat is trimmed with scissors while the deep plane travels on the superficial cervical fascia under the platysma muscle (**Fig. 5**).

If subplatysmal fat is bulgy, we elevate the anterior part of the platysma muscle using 2 Alice clamps; we tangentially excise the trapezoid deep fat until we reach the level of anterior belly of the digastric muscle. We seldom need partial resection of the anterior belly of digastric muscle because the over-resection of fat creates a characteristic deepening of the frontal part of the neck, which gives the impression of a gunshot deformity.

How does the presence of visible platysma muscle bands alter your approach? Do you undermine, plicate, transect, and partially resect platysmal muscle bands?

To address thin soft bands in a young neck, a lateral fixation to Lore's and mastoid fascia anchoring points is usually enough, providing a good satisfaction rate to our patients (**Figs. 6–13**).

When we have to deal with multiple or hard bands, we think it is highly important to evaluate the platysma muscles diastasis in the midline. We usually suture it using 4.0 polydioxanone sutures by performing invagination of the medial

Fig. 6. First patient, before picture, jowls and midface laxity.

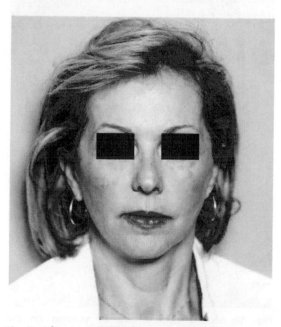

Fig. 7. After high SMAS face and neck lift.

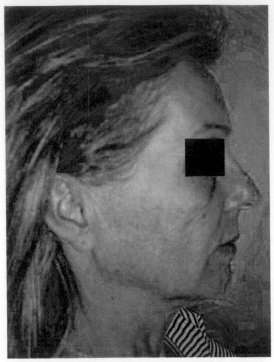

Fig. 8. Jowls protruding from the mandibular angle.

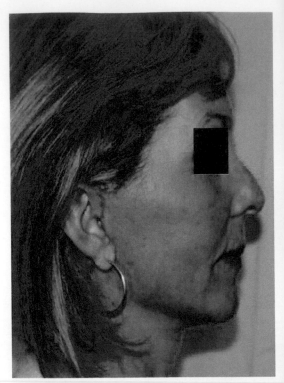

Fig. 9. Facial contour corrected.

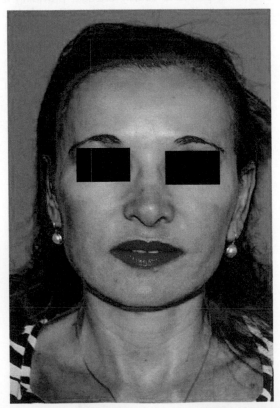

Fig. 10. Second patient, loss of volume on the zygoma, fulness on the lower third of the face.

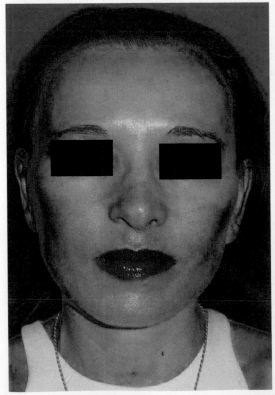

Fig. 11. Correction of the deformities with no aditional filling.

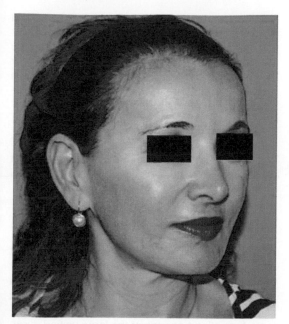

Fig. 12. Facial contour undefined.

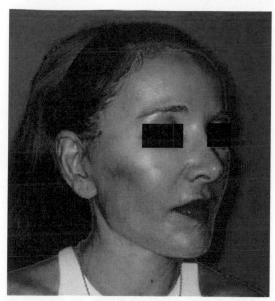

Fig. 13. Cervicomandibular angle with definition.

aspect of platysma muscle and a back cut in the area above the cricoid. When dealing with multiple bands on fatty necks, a boomerang incision of the platysma is appropriate, which connects the lower part of platysma muscle with the previously elevated flap in front of the sternocleidomastoid muscle. This maneuver provides better definition and less contracture of the neck. We begin with

small bites from the mastoid fascia up to the proximal third of the mandible in order to avoid any damage to the marginal mandibular branch, using 4.0 nylon sutures. This surgical manipulation

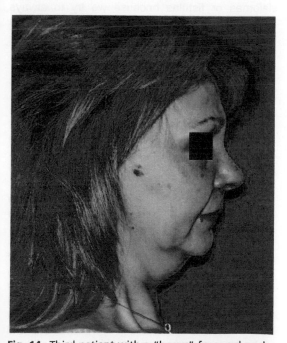

Fig. 14. Third patient with a "heavy" face and neck.

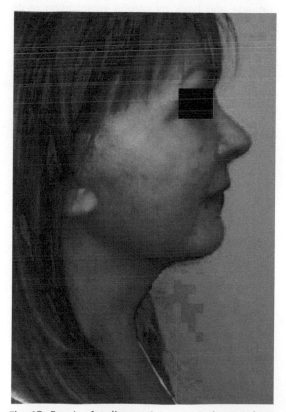

Fig. 15. Result after liposuction, corset platymaplasty and ancoring to Lore's fascia.

achieves the goal of improving and supporting the definition of the mandible. A corset platysmaplasty may be combined with all of the aforementioned procedures depending on the extent of the problem in the initial phase (**Figs. 14** and **15**).

Discuss Submaxillary Gland Reduction

Submandibular glands rarely require treatment because they do not disrupt the neck contour by lying deep to the plane tangent to the inferior border of the mandible and the ipsilateral anterior belly of the digastric muscle. We are trying to treat them through the additional support of the corset platysmaplasty because their partial or total excision is associated with numerous complications.

Do you partially resect the anterior bellies of the digastric muscles?

Yes we do. If their hypertrophy is significant enough to alter the neck angle, we perform an anterior digastric myectomy using forceps and electrocautery; we divide the muscle near the mandible and the hyoid (**Fig. 16**). We usually achieve satisfactory neck contouring by just removing a small part of the belly (about one-third); after meticulous hemostasis, we approximate the platysma muscle down to the cricoid cartilage and back by careful invagination of its edges.

Do you think there is a need to drain necks?

Soft silicone Blake-type drains are routinely placed subcutaneously bilaterally under low negative pressure with exit ports in the occipital hair-bearing skin. We think they add to the dissected neck flap adherence and, as long as negative pressure stays low, they cannot compromise flap

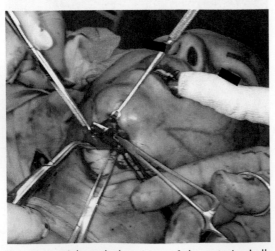

Fig. 16. Partial surgical excision of the anterior belly of the digastric muscle.

viability. Drain tubes must be flat, though, to avoid additional pressure to the overlying postauricular thin dermal flap. Drains are kept for 24 to 48 hours (depending on the amount of drainage per 24 hours), and special care is given to always place a drain in the cavity created by the subplatysmal fat or anterior digastric belly excision.

Do you use fibrin glue in the neck?

Even though we are familiar with the fibrin glue–low skin tension technique, we have not used it yet in our patients, even though its use is well established.

SEQUELAE AND COMPLICATIONS

We advise smokers to stop smoking at least 30 days before the date of operation, and we treat their necks with less aggressive dissection and tension in our anchoring techniques. A neck lift following a facelift is prone to seroma or hematoma formation because of the large unified surgical fields. We do not apply compressive garments on the skin, and we avoid skin-resurfacing procedures in combination with our neck lift. In the case of seroma formation, we treat it with transdermal evacuation. Hematoma formation led one of our patients back to the operating theater 4 hours after the procedure concluded for further hemostatic management. One female patient presented postauricular skin slough with partial necrosis (smoker), which healed remarkably well by secondary intention. We have not encountered any sialomas or fistulas because we try to always keep parotid glands covered. We do not use dressings in our face and neck rejuvenation procedures, except for an initial coverage with Steri-Strips (3M, St Paul, MN) on the submental area.

The effect of residual skin sloughing responds excellently to energy-based noninvasive techniques; closed liposuction in an outpatient basis is able to correct minor postoperative localized areas of lipodystrophy. Postliposuction submental edema, when severe, requires compression garments and massage for several weeks to fully resolve.

Recurrent or residual hard muscle bands can be treated with closed myotomies using the SurgiWire technique (MicroAire Aesthetics, Charlottesville, VA), a nokor needle, or cauterization with an insulated tip. Chemical denervation with 10 units of botulinum toxin A in each band is enough for active bands and must be repeated accordingly. Special absorbable cone-shaped sutures can be placed in any postoperative stage in order to achieve a better mandibular border definition. When lateral platysma fixation does not provide adequate lifting, we can always return under local anesthesia and plicate the platysma in the midline through a small submental incision after 6 to 9 months.

Because all of our neck rejuvenation techniques do not rely on skin strength to provide long-lasting results (Video 1), we have not encountered any severe wound healing complications, like hypertrophic scars or keloids. (We routinely perform surgery on Caucasian patients.) Close scar observation during the first postoperative month is mandatory to optimize wound healing and secure a satisfactory aesthetic outcome.

SUPPLEMENTARY DATA

Supplementary data related to this article can be found online at http://dx.doi.org/10.1016/j.cps.2013.09.008.

REFERENCES

1. Baker DC. Minimal incision rhytidectomy (short scar face lift) with lateral SMASectomy. Aesthet Surg J 2001;21:68–79.
2. Mitz V, Peyronie M. The superficial musculoaponeurotic system (SMAS) in the parotid and cheek area. Plast Reconstr Surg 1976;58:80–8.
3. Connell BF, Gaon A. Surgical correction of aesthetic contour problems of the neck. Clin Plast Surg 1983; 10:491.
4. Furnas DW. The retaining ligaments of the cheek. Plast Reconstr Surg 1989;83:11.
5. Loré JM Jr. 2nd edition. An atlas of head and neck surgery, vol. 2. Philadelpia: Saunders; 1973. p. 596–7.
6. Labbé D, Franco RG, Nicolas J. Platysma suspension and platysmaplasty during neck-lift and analysis of 30 cases. Plast Reconstr Surg 2006;117:2001.
7. Jost G, Levet Y. Parotid fascia and face-lifting: a critical evaluation of the SMAS concept. Plast Reconstr Surg 1984;74:42.
8. Jones BM, Grover R, Hamilton S. The efficacy of surgical drainage in cervicofacial rhytidectomy: a prospective, randomized, controlled trial. Plast Reconstr Surg 2007;120:263–70.
9. Daher JC. Closed platysmotomy: a new procedure for the treatment of platysma bands without skin dissection. Aesthetic Plast Surg 2011;35: 866–77.
10. Shah AR, Rosenberg D. Defining the facial extent of the platysma muscle. Review of 71 consecutive face-lifts. Arch Facial Plast Surg 2009;11(6): 405–8.
11. Panfilov DE. MIDI face-lift and tricuspidal SMAS-flap. Aesthetic Plast Surg 2003;27:27–37.
12. Zoumalan R, Rizk SS. Hematoma rates in drainless deep-plane face-lift surgery with and without the use of fibrin glue. Arch Facial Plast Surg 2008; 10(2):103–7.
13. Graivier M. Wire subcision for complete release of depressions, subdermal attachments, and scars. Aesthet Surg J 2006;26:387–94.
14. Gamboa GM, Vasconez LO. Suture suspension technique for mid face and neck rejuvenation. Ann Plast Surg 2009;62:478–81.
15. De Benito J, Pizzamiglio R, Theodorou D, et al. Facial rejuvenation and improvement of malar projection using sutures with absorbable cones: surgical technique and case series. Aesthetic Plast Surg 2011;35:248–53.

Restoring the Neck Contour

Claudio Cardoso De Castro, MD*,
Jose Horacio Aboudib, MD, Antônia Márcia Cupello, MD,
Ana Claudia Roxo, MD

KEYWORDS

- Neck contour • Restoring • Neck deformity • Rhytidoplasty

KEY POINTS

- To restore neck contour, we do not favor the following procedures: Submandibular gland resections: Operations on the submandibular gland may yield severe complications, and the benefits are not worth the risk. Digastric muscle operations: We see no advantages to operations on the digastric muscles. They are masticatory muscles.
- To provide the best outcome for the patient, the surgeon must respect the complexity and variance of neck defects, the limitations of each case, and the surgeon's own limitations.

Editor Commentary: Claudio had the opportunity to dissect dozens of cadavers and as a result of this important study, he described the three typical anatomic appearances and the associated decussation of the platysma muscles. In this chapter he takes us through his personal evolution in necklifting based upon the clinical findings and working towards a desirable clinical outcome. Even Claudio's relatively simple maneuver of adding 1cm to the submental incision has been helpful in allowing improved vision to the relevant submental anatomy with no consequence in patient satisfaction.

A neck deformity is the main complaint of patients who seek a rhytidoplasty. Patients present with diverse ages, different deformities, and variable aspirations, which brings a tough challenge for the surgeon.

Observing **Fig. 1**, the differences among patients are noticeable, showing variable deformities, such as skin excess, fat amount and distribution, bone structure, and so forth. Therefore, it is mandatory to provide a very personal surgical plan for each one.

Skin excess together with fat and muscle superficial muscular aponeurotic system (SMAS)/platysma alterations are responsible for neck contour deformities. These alterations will be more or less noticeable according to the bone structure, skin quality, position of hyoid bone, and the submandibular gland. According to the magnitude of these factors, the surgical plan is aimed at the elimination/attenuation of the deformities. To plan the procedure appropriately, one must

respect the limitations of each case and even the surgeon's limitations.

We do not favor submandibular gland resection and/or digastric muscle operations. The operations on the submandibular gland may yield severe complications, and the benefits are not worth the risk. We do not see the advantages of operations on the digastric muscles. They are masticatory muscles.

In most of the cases, we unite the skin dissection at the suprahyoid region.

We open the submental area whenever there is alteration at the median line. In doubt, we always open it. We never regretted opening the neck; in some cases, we would have had a better result if we had opened the neck. It is important to state that we never had a complaint on the imperceptible scar below the chin.

When there is severe deformity in the jaw line, we recommend an ample SMAS dissection.

When lipectomies are performed, they are done so in a limited fashion in order to avoid

Plastic Surgery Service, University of the State of Rio De Janeiro, Rio De Janeiro, Brasil
* Corresponding author. Rua Domingos Ferreira, 140/301, Copacabana, Rio De Janeiro 22050010, Brasil.
E-mail address: cdecastro@uol.com.br

Clin Plastic Surg 41 (2014) 51–56
http://dx.doi.org/10.1016/j.cps.2013.09.012
0094-1298/14/$ – see front matter © 2014 Elsevier Inc. All rights reserved.

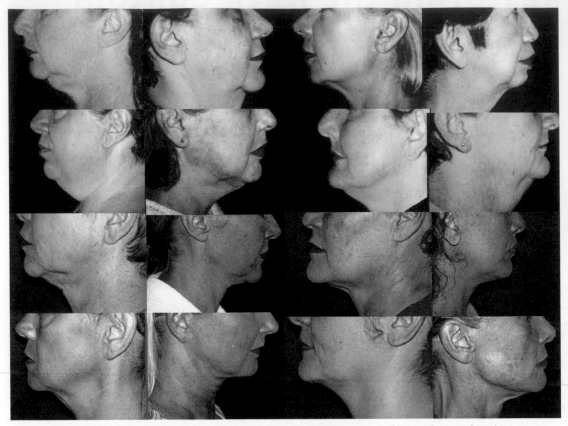

Fig. 1. Different types of patients showing the variation of the alterations of lower face and neck.

skin retractions or artificial results and skin undulations.

For submental aspiration, we use Pontes cannula (**Fig. 1**) that, in our opinion, facilitates the fat removal evenly, in an open manner. We do not favor subplatysmal defatting because there is a natural space between the platysma muscle and the mylohyoid muscle. If fat is removed, the muscles will heal and a deformity will occur that is very difficult to correct.

When fat is removed, the medial fibers of the platysma muscles are dissected to evaluate the thickness, anatomic behavior, and flaccidity of the muscles. A lateral dissection is done, and the muscle excess is carefully observed and removed. A medial suture is performed following a medial section as described by Aston using scissors as proposed by Aboudib. For us, it is extremely important to remove the muscle in excess because the approximation of the medial fibers in a great percentage of patients with muscle excess will show redundancy of the muscle if it is not reduced (**Fig. 2**). That is why there is much importance to knowing and understanding the anatomic knowledge of the anatomy of the medial fibers of the platysma muscle.

SOME REMARKS ON THE ANATOMY OF MEDIAL FIBERS OF PLATYSMA MUSCLE

In 1980, we published an article on platysma anatomy where we dissected 100 formalized cadavers.[1–24] The initial purpose of the study was to observe the mandibular ramus of the facial nerve. When we were studying the photographs, we noticed different types of distribution of the medial fibers of the platysma muscle in the midline. We noticed the fibers were joined or

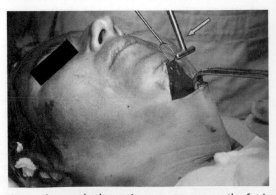

Fig. 2. The canula the authors use to remove the fat in the neck. It has 3 holes and a form of "T."

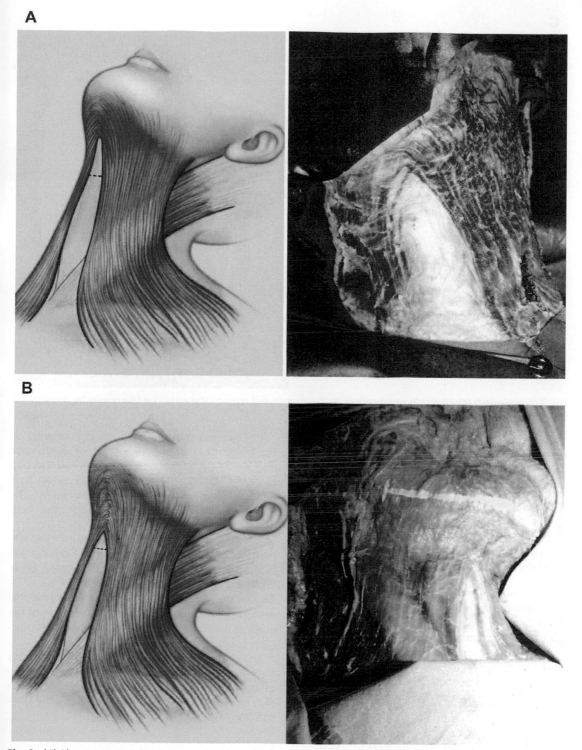

Fig. 3. (*A*) Platysma type I fibers decussate about 3 cm below the chin being more separated or less separated at the suprahyoid region. (*B*) Platysma type II fibers are joined at the submental region behaving as a single muscle.

C

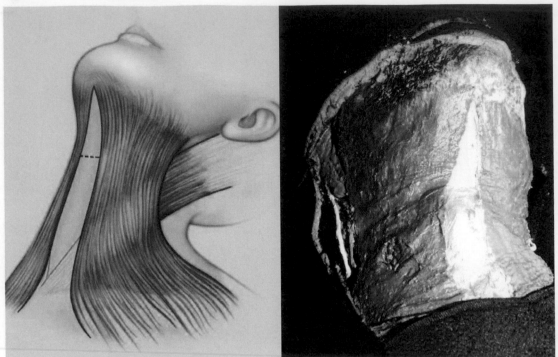

Fig. 3. (*continued*) (*C*) Fibers do not interlace at the suprahyoid region. The muscular fibers may be more or less separated presenting different grades of thickness.

separated. Then we classified the fibers into 3 different groups.

1. Type I: The fibers interlace 1 to 2 cm below the chin (**Fig. 3**A).
2. Type II: The fibers interlace at thyroid's cartilage level behaving as a single muscle at the suprahyoid region (**Fig. 3**B).
3. Type III: The fibers do not interlace. They go straight to the chin (**Fig. 3**C).

The importance of this knowledge is to keep in mind whether or not these fibers are found separated. They can be more or less separated, presenting variable grades of flaccidity and also different grades of thickness. This variability led us to evaluate the grade of muscle excess when treating neck deformities because if you do not pay attention to this, in many patients, flaccidity will remain.

SMAS

Concerning treatment of the SMAS, plication, SMASectomy, and dissection more or less extended are the choices. The extension varies according to the deformity of each case. We like to dissect SMAS because we can mobilize the tissues, repositioning them according to the anatomic findings.

The extension of the undermining depends on the magnitude of the alteration of each case and when the dissection is performed the flap is being pulled, the surgeon feels when it is enough for that patient. For the jowls, the standard SMAS undermining yields the best results.

A submental incision is performed in most patients (about 80%). This incision is a 4-cm incision located 3 to 4 mm behind the submental crease. We used to do a 3-cm incision; but a 0.5-cm increase at each extremity meant nothing to the final result, and it helps a lot in the visualization of the surgical field as well as the manipulation of the surgical tools.

The retroauricular incision may stop just behind the earlobe (Baker) or at the level of the ear implantation into the occipital area; or in cases when the skin excess is great, the incision follows the hairline (**Fig. 4**).

COMPLICATIONS

As in any surgical procedure, complications can occur, such as hematomas, nerve injury (most commonly the mandibular ramus), skin necrosis, keloid formation, hypertrophic scar, skin irregularities, infection, and dissatisfaction.

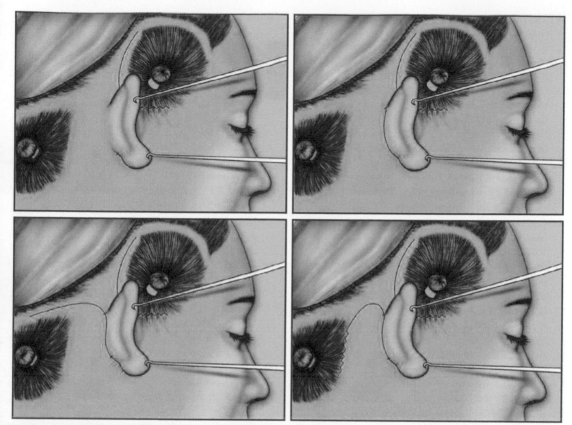

Fig. 4. The options for retroauricular incisions.

Mandibular ramus nerve injury is usually caused by liposuction or cauterization. Commonly, the recovery occurs in 1 to 3 months.

Skin necrosis may be the result of superficial undermining of the skin, heavy smoking (both active and passive), and excess traction on the skin.

Skin irregularities are usually caused by defatting. They also may occur from a hematoma that was not well treated.

Infection is extremely rare; the are several causes, such as teeth inflammation, not properly performed asepsis, and so forth.

Unsatisfied patients is an issue that is extremely difficult to manage. Patients who have had very well-performed procedures and are unhappy sometimes become extremely difficult to take care of at our offices.

When it is necessary to perform a revision, we advise waiting 1 year before performing any secondary procedures.

SUMMARY

As discussed, we deal with different kinds of patients exhibiting different anatomic arrangements of the structures in their neck, different ages, and different expectations; and there are several techniques from which to choose. We must have successful results in every single case. Patients have no idea of the deformity they show. They demand a fast recovery with the best possible result that is long lasting.

Because of the diversity of the involved elements, a neck lift turns out to be an extremely complex challenge for the surgeon, demanding both an accurate technique and common sense.

In summary, it is not easy to define a difficult neck or to evaluate the result solely as the operating surgeon. The result will define it; depending on the patient, she or he will evaluate the result and state whether he or she is pleased or is dissatisfied with the result.

REFERENCES

1. Cardoso de Castro C. Extensive cervical and lower face lipectomy: its importance and anatomical basis. Ann Plast Surg 1980;4(5):370–5.
2. Cardoso de Castro C. The anatomy of platysma muscle. Plast Reconstr Surg 1980;66(5):680–3.
3. Cardoso de Castro C. Extensive mandibular and cervical lipectomy. Aesthetic Plast Surg 1981;5(3): 239–48.

4. Cardoso de Castro C. The value of the anatomical classification of the medial fibers of platysma muscle in cervical lifting. Transactions of the VIIIth International Congress of Plastic and Reconstructive Surgery. Montreal, 1983. p. 515–6.

5. Cardoso de Castro C. The value of the anatomical study of the platysma muscle in cervical lifting. Aesthetic Plast Surg 1984;8(11):7–11.

6. Cardoso de Castro C. Superficial musculoaponeurotic system-platysma: a continuous study. Ann Plast Surg 1991;26(3):201–11.

7. Cardoso de Castro C. Treatment of deformities of the neck and lower third of the face. Operative tech oculoplastic, orbital. Reconstr Surg 1999;2(3):123–30.

8. Cardoso de Castro C. The changing role of platysma in face lifting. Plast Reconstr Surg 2000; 150(2):764–75.

9. Cardoso de Castro C. Anatomy of the neck and procedure selection. Clin Plast Surg 2008;35(4): 625–42.

10. Baker DC. Face lift with submandibular gland and digastric muscle resection. Radical neck rhytidectomy. Aesthet Surg J 2006;26:85–92.

11. Aston JS. Platysma-SMAS cervical rhytidoplasty. Clin Plast Surg 1983;10:507–20.

12. Baker DC. Lateral SMASectomy. Plast Reconstr Surg 1997;100:509–20.

13. Baker DC. Minimal incision rhytidectomy (short scar face lift) with lateral SMASectomy: evolution and application. Aesthet Surg J 2001;21:14–26.

14. Feldmann JJ. Corset platysmaplasty. Plast Reconstr Surg 1990;85:333–43.

15. Pitanguy I. Facial cosmetic surgery: a 30-year perspective. Plast Reconstr Surg 2000;105:1527.

16. Barton FE Jr. Rhytidectomy and the nasolabial fold. Plast Reconstr Surg 1992;90:601.

17. Connell BC. The value of platysma muscle flaps. Ann Plast Surg 1978;1:34.

18. Peterson RA. The role of the platysma muscle in cervical lifting. In: Em Goulian P, Courtis E, editors. Symposium of surgery of the aging face. St Louis (MO): Mosby; 1978. p. 115–24.

19. Aston SJ. Platysma muscle in rhytidoplasty. Ann Plast Surg 1979;3:529.

20. Mitz V, Peyronie M. The superficial musculoaponeurotic system (SMAS) in the parotid and cheek area. Plast Reconstr Surg 1976;58:80.

21. Millard DR, Garst WP, Beck RL, et al. Submental and submandibular lipectomy in conjunction with a face lift, in the male or female. Plast Reconstr Surg 1972; 49:385.

22. Badin J. Rejuvenescimento facial - Nova técnica de lipectomia submaxilar e submentoniana. Rev Bras Cir 1972;62:99.

23. Pitanguy I, Pamplona DC, Giuntini ME, et al. Computational simulation of rhytidectomy by the round lifting technique. Rev Bras Cir 1995;85: 213–8.

24. Pontes R. Extended dissection of the mental area in face-lifts. Ann Plast Surg 1991;27:439–56.

Open Neck Contouring

Daniel Labbé, MD[a],*, Jean-Philippe Giot, MD[b]

KEYWORDS

- Open neck • Contouring • Technique • Complications • Neck lift • Digastric corset
- Anterior approach • Platysma • Lateral repositioning

KEY POINTS

- Lateral platysma repositioning (platysma suspension) using the first crease of the neck platysma key point alone or together with/submental approach to rebuilt the floor of the mouth using the digastric corset after subplatysma fat resection and the retaining ligaments between platysma, digastric and mylohyoïd muscle are rebuilt in the subhyoïd area/running barbed sutures are used.

Editor Commentary: I met Daniel on several occasions and, while lecturing in Guadalajara for the annual Jose Guerrosantos Symposium, Daniel discussed his approach to rejuvenating the neck utilizing his "digastric corset" technique which I was unaware of. This chapter presents his logical approach to surgery of the aging neck including this novel approach to the submental area. I asked him and his co-author, Jean-Plilippe to describe the digastric corset since it appears frequently in his chapter.

INTRODUCTION

We published in 2013 the technique of the digastric corset. We started from the observations of patients who were operated upon with platysma suspension and did not present with satisfying results in the submental area. Platysma bands were sometimes visible and in bulky necks the overall result was insufficient. We went to the anatomy laboratory and studied the anchorage of the platysma and the digastric muscles relative to the floor of the mouth. We found a retaining ligament between the anterior digastric bellies and the mylohyoid muscle which restricts the displacement of the anterior belly of the digastric laterally but no longitudinally. The platysma is adherent to the inferior aspect of the digastric muscle and through it to the floor of the mouth explaining some of the insufficiency of the lateral rhytidectomy approach in the area between the two anterior bellies of the digastric muscles.

The digastric corset is a running suture of the digastric-to-mylohyoid retaining ligament, performed through a small retro-chin incision after interdigastric fat removal. The medial displacement

of the digastric fills the interdigastric fat hollow, tightens the floor of the mouth and displaces the platysma medial insertion. A second platysmal corset is performed to close the dead space and further lighten the anterior neck. The submaxillary gland is moved upward in a platysmal hammock, which avoids a specific procedure. The combination of digastric corset and cervico-facial rhytidectomy gives synergistic effects in the rejuvenation of the anterior neck with very good restoration of the anterior cervical angle even in cases of bulky necks (grade IV of Knize neck cosmetic deformities).

WHAT INCISION(S) DO YOU TYPICALLY USE IN THE THIN NECK AND THE HEAVY NECK IN BOTH YOUNG AND OLDER PATIENTS?

For moderate alteration of neck contour in thin necks (Knize grade I and II), we perform a cervico-facial rhytidectomy with lateral platysma suspension.[1] The incisions are those of classic facial rhytidectomy. Briefly, it starts in the hairs in the temple area with a stairlike broken line, in the pre-auricular sulcus down to the superior part of the

---

[a] Private Practice, 4, Place Fontette, 14000 Caen, France; [b] Division of Plastic Surgery, Department of Surgery, Centre Hospitalier de l'Université deMontréal, Montréal, Canada
* Corresponding author.
E-mail address: dr.labbe@wanadoo.fr

Clin Plastic Surg 41 (2014) 57–63
http://dx.doi.org/10.1016/j.cps.2013.09.014
0094-1298/14/$ – see front matter © 2014 Elsevier Inc. All rights reserved.

tragus, on the free edge of the tragus down to the intertragal sulcus, around the ear lobe, in the retro-auricular sulcus, and in front of the hairline horizontally, at the largest part of the auricle (**Fig. 1**A). Once in the hairs, the line is drawn upward for a few more centimeters, which hides the scar better, as suggested by Daniel Marchac (see **Fig. 1**B).

If medial platysma cords are not perfectly corrected by the clinical simulation test, meaning that the platysma is adherent to the digastric muscles and cannot be moved by a lateral suspension, we add a digastric corset.[2]

In young heavy necks, we perform an anterior neck approach alone. Isolated liposuction is reserved for a small deformity when fat is located electively in a subcutaneous position. If fat is accumulated in an interdigastric position, we perform a liposuction, digastric corset (where this fat is resected), and large skin undermining laterally to redistribute the skin excess of the midline to the submandibular area.

In older heavy necks, the neck approach is the same, but we also perform a lateral platysma suspension.

WHAT ARE YOUR INDICATIONS FOR LIMITING YOUR ACCESS INCISIONS TO THE SUBMENTAL AREA OR THE LATERAL APPROACH? IN WHICH CASES DO YOU USE BOTH INCISIONS?

We perform a lateral incision solely in cases in which clinical simulation of platysma suspension

completely restores the anterior cervical angle using patient pictures (**Fig. 2**).

Young people complain that the anterior cervical angle, without aging signs, is an anatomic abnormality. A clinical observation might be an association of interdigastric fat hypertrophy, digastric malposition, floor of the mouth ptosis, or accumulated fat in subcutaneous tissue. Only in these cases do we perform an anterior cervical approach, sometimes under local anesthesia, without facial rhytidectomy.

In all other cases, with a mix of anatomic abnormalities and aging, we use a combined lateral and submental approach.

WHAT IS YOUR APPROACH TO DEFATTING THE NECK? WHICH FATTY LAYERS DO YOU RESECT (IE, SUBCUTANEOUS, INTERPLATYSMAL, SUBPLATYSMAL FAT)? WHAT ROLE DOES LIPOSUCTION PLAY IN YOUR TECHNIQUE, EITHER ALONE OR IN COMBINATION WITH OPEN TECHNIQUES?

We use liposuction to defat the subcutaneous and interplatysmal layers. We perform a liposuction when a pinch test of the neck tissues shows a thickness of 1 cm or more. We do not use other defatting methods because liposuction is reliable and has an extremely low morbidity in this anatomic area. We begin the surgical procedure after infiltration of an epinephrine serum solution (1 mgm of epinephrine for 1 L of infusate serum).

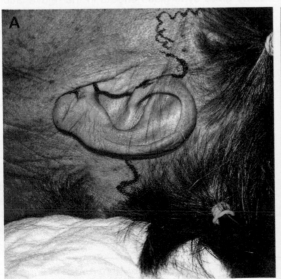
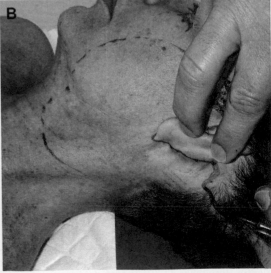

Fig. 1. (*A*) The preincision marking starts in the hairs in the temple area with a stairlike broken line, in the preauricular sulcus down to the superior part of the tragus, on the free edge of the tragus down to the intertragal sulcus, and around the ear lobe. (*B*) The line is placed in the retroauricular sulcus and in front of the hairline goes horizontally and then upward for a few more centimeters.

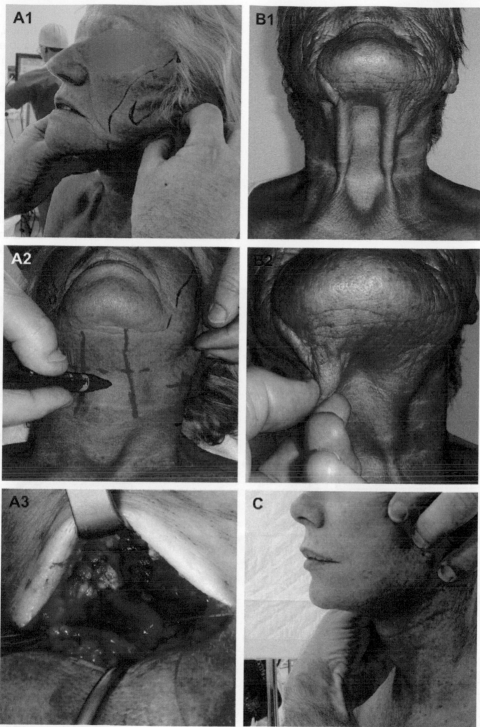

Fig. 2. (*A1*) Clinical simulation of a platysma suspension procedure shows an incomplete restoration of the anterior neck contours, especially in the submental area. Blue images represent the area of skin flap undermining and the superior key point of platysma suspension. (*A2*) While the patient is lying on their back, further landmarks are drawn (*red*): anterior digastric bellies and platysma bands, lower key point of platysma suspension (*cross*). (*A3*) The anterior approach of the neck starts with a 4-cm-long incision 2 mm behind the retrochin sulcus, which makes skin undermining easy to perform. The chin is held with a hook, a Farabeuf retracts the neck skin, allowing the next steps, which consist of platysma incision, interdigastric fat removal, and digastric corset (here with a 3/0 barbed suture). (*B1*) This patient shows an aged neck with marked platysma bands. (*B2*) Cutaneous pinch test confirmed a low subcutaneous fat deposit. For this patient, a cervicofacial rhytidectomy and digastric corset were proposed. (*C*) In this 50-year-old woman, clinical simulation of platysma suspension shows good restoration of the anterior neck.

Cases in which subcutaneous fat alone is thickened are rare; in most cases, the volume of interdigastric fat has also increased. The clinical test of F. Nahai is particularly useful to assess the volume of the subcutaneous and the interdigastric fat, which we treat by a direct excision followed by a digastric corset.[3]

HOW DOES THE PRESENCE OF VISIBLE PLATYSMA MUSCLE BANDS ALTER YOUR APPROACH? DO YOU UNDERMINE, PLICATE, TRANSECT, PARTIALLY RESECT, BACK CUT, AND SO FORTH, PLATYSMAL MUSCLE BANDS?

We do not resect or transect the platysma. Visible platysma bands might be considered in 2 parts in the submandibular area. The lateral bands, which are located above the submaxillary gland and the sternocleidomastoid in the background, and are well treated by platysma suspension.

Medial platysma bands are above the anterior belly of the digastric muscles, where they are firmly adherent. In some cases, depending on patient platysma anatomy, medial bands are not correctly treated by platysma suspension. We perform a digastric corset (**Fig. 3**) to reconstruct the floor of the mouth followed by a platysmal corset, which tightens the whole submandibular area medially, in association with the platysma suspension, which tightens laterally. Medial platysma bands are therefore attached to the floor of the mouth, which is located well above the preoperative state.

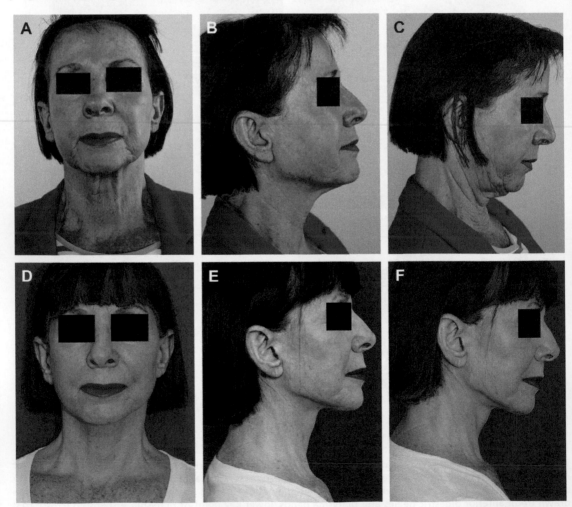

Fig. 3. (*A*) This 69-year-old woman presented principally with neck platysma bands and skin laxity. (*B*) Holding the head to the right, platysma bands alter the anterior cervical angle. (*C*) While tilting the head, major alterations in the anterior neck appear, caused by the aging of skin, platysma bands, and digastric malposition. (*D*) A facelift, platysma suspension, and digastric corset were performed, showing great improvement in the cervical angle. (*E*) The procedure restored the mandibular contour and the visibility of the laryngotracheal structures. (*F*) In particular, the jowl drop and submaxillary gland ptosis were well corrected while tilting the head.

To further improve the results, if platysma bands are extremely prominent, we use botulinum neurotoxin to rest the platysma during surgery and healing.

SUBMAXILLARY GLAND REDUCTION

We never perform submaxillary gland reduction, because the hammock created by the combination of digastric corset and platysma suspension corrects the ptosis of the submaxillary gland, with extremely low morbidity (**Fig. 4**).

DO YOU PARTIALLY RESECT THE ANTERIOR BELLIES OF THE DIGASTRIC MUSCLES?

We previously performed partial resection of the anterior bellies of the digastric muscles before we found the digastric corset. This new procedure corrects the ptosis of the floor of the mouth and the protruding bellies of the digastric muscles.

With an extremely low complication rate, 1 case of lymphedema in 20 patients, and given the good results obtained by digastric corset, this discourages us from performing partial resection of the digastric muscles (**Fig. 5**).

DO YOU BELIEVE THERE IS A NEED TO DRAIN NECKS?

With the procedures that we use (cervicofacial rhytidectomy, liposuction, interdigastric fat removal, and digastric corset), we do not drain necks if all dead spaces are closed. Interdigastric space is completely closed by the digastric corset. Platysma bands are sutured to the anterior bellies of the digastric muscles, thereafter closing the remaining space. We do not drain liposuction. We use a drain only under the facial skin flap laterally, which we believe could be abandoned in favor of quilting sutures.

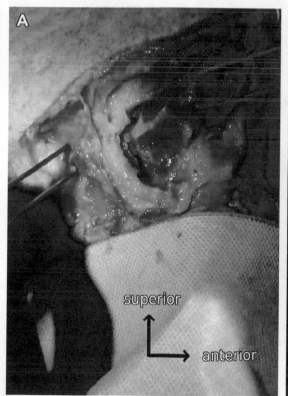
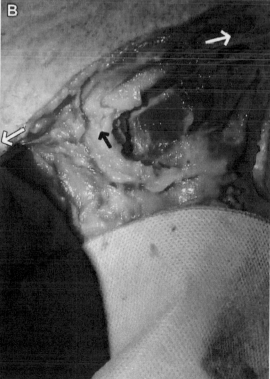

Fig. 4. Anatomic dissection of the neck, side aspect. (*A*) Before applying any tension on the tissues, the submaxillary gland is positioned low. (*B*) When the digastric corset (medial displacement of the anterior belly of the digastric muscle) and platysma suspension are simulated by forceps (*white arrows*), the submaxillary gland (*black arrow*) and the intermediate tendon of the digastric muscle are moved superiorly.

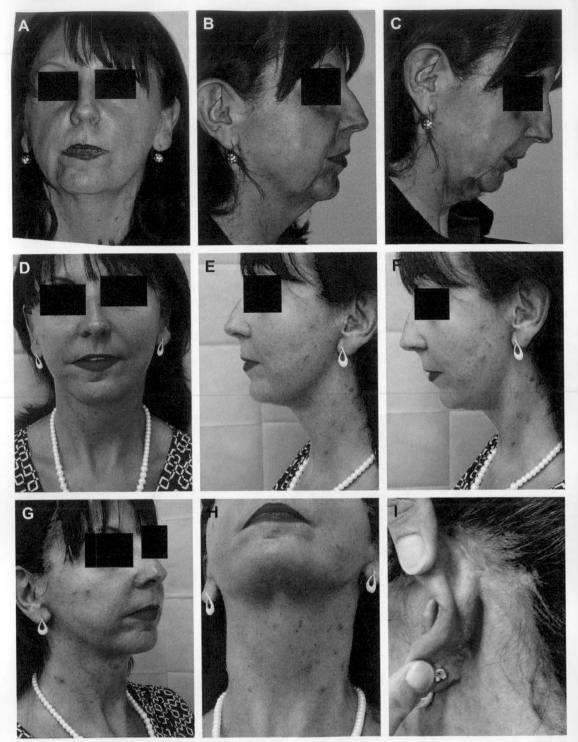

Fig. 5. (*A*) This patient complained about facial aging and especially of jaw drop and cervical deformities. (*B*) This patient's clinical examination revealed IV Knize cosmetic grade alteration of the anterior neck, which was not fully restored by a platysma suspension clinical test. (*C*) The patient complained of neck deformities on flexion. (*D*) We performed a cervicofacial rhytidectomy, digastric corset, and platysma suspension, with a good result on the visibility of the mandibular edge. (*E*) A lateral aspect shows good restoration of the anterior cervical angle. (*F*) The submandibular area is well defined, with clear delineation of the sternocleidomastoid muscle. (*G*) The correction of the submaxillary gland ptosis is satisfying without any other surgical procedure. (*H*) The retrochin scar is discreet, and the restoration of Ellenbogen esthetic criteria of a youthful neck are met.[5] (*I*) The retroauricular scar is well hidden behind the largest part of the auricle.

DO YOU USE FIBRIN GLUE IN THE NECK?

We do not use fibrin glue because undermining is limited. Also, a study[4] found that fibrin glue did not significantly change the occurrence of edema and ecchymosis in facelifts.

EXPECTED SEQUELAE OF YOUR TECHNIQUE AND COMPLICATIONS THAT YOU HAVE OBSERVED AND HOW YOU TREATED THEM

The feeling of submental tightening is treated by myorelaxant (tetrazepam) for 6 days.

In a series of 20 patients, we had only 1 small lymphedema, which was assessed by ultrasonography. We injected a small amount of corticoids and asked the patient to stop self-massages. A larger lymphedema would be treated by a surgical procedure to close the dead spaces. This complication is prevented by applying compression to the submandibular area with tape (micropore) or with a facelift compression garment for eight days.

We were accustomed to treating a medial hollow after liposuction by fat grafting. Since we have begun performing the digastric corset, we have not observed a medial hollow after interdigastric fat resection, because the anterior bellies of the digastric muscles are displaced medially and fill the dead space.

TIMING FOR ANY REVISIONS OF A NECK LIFT

If needed, we perform a revision procedure at 6 months after the first surgery. We perform a digastric corset in patients who do not present a large and bulky neck to stabilize the results of a facelift.

REFERENCES

1. Labbé D, Franco RG, Nicolas J. Platysma suspension and platysmaplasty during neck lift: anatomical study and analysis of 30 cases. Plast Reconstr Surg 2006;117(6):2001–7 [discussion: 2008–10].
2. Labbé D, Giot JP, Kaluzinski E. Submental area rejuvenation by digastric corset: anatomical study and clinical application in 20 cases. Aesthetic Plast Surg 2013;37(2):222–31.
3. Mejia JD, Nahai FR, Nahai F, et al. Isolated management of the aging neck. Semin Plast Surg 2009; 23(4):264–73.
4. Marchac D, Greensmith AL. Early postoperative efficacy of fibrin glue in face lifts: a prospective randomized trial. Plast Reconstr Surg 2005;115(3): 911–6 [discussion: 917–8].
5. Ellenbogen R, Karlin JV. Visual criteria for success in restoring the youthful neck. Plast Reconstr Surg 1980;66(6):826–37.

The LOPP—Lateral Overlapping Plication of the Platysma
An Effective Neck Lift Without Submental Incision

Raul Gonzalez, MD

KEYWORDS

- Neck lift • Cervicoplasty • Platysma • Submandibular gland • Jawline • Mandibular angle
- Lateral plication • LOPP

KEY POINTS

- Lateral plication of the platysma, when following some essential rules, can substitute with advantages for medial plication in all cases, no matter the severity of the case.
- Lateral overlapping plication of the platysma (LOPP) is done by a linear opening on the platysma muscle, over a line indicated by the second premolar tooth and strongly overlapping the muscular edges of the incision.
- Mild submandibular gland ptosis is treated by muscular overlapping, which tightens the platysma over the gland, pushing it up.
- Partial resection of the submandibular gland is done easily and safely through the LOPP platysma incision.
- LOPP has advantages over medial line plication: it Is Incisionless, is less undermining, treats submandibular gland bumps prophylactically, provides easy and safe access to submandibular gland, and needs less defatting.

Editor Commentary: *While teaching in Brazil, I had the pleasure to reunite with Raul. It was then that he described his approach to the neck which I found fascinating. His submandibular lateral approach to the platysma muscle and the submaxillary gland is a departure from the other authors' techniques and is worth considering when the anatomy and the well described technical steps are followed. I was excited to see Raul's impressive results in neck contouring achieved without a submental incision.*

THE LOPP NECK LIFTING
Incisions

By adopting the LOPP method, surgeons abandon the submental incision, which is never necessary with the LOOP neck lift. The entire approach to the neck is done through the lateral access. Surgeons can use the incision used routinely. I usually begin an incision below the sideburn on the temporal area; then, the incision follows the border of the tragus and on the retroauricular area comes downward on the hairline for a small segment and finishes inside the hair (**Fig. 1**). The posterior incision can be shorter in younger people, but short incisions, finishing just posteriorly above the ear lobule, as short scars style, usually are not enough to take off the large excess of skin resulting from the procedure.

Department of Surgery, Medicine School of UNAERP, Universidade de Ribeirao Preto, 661 Amadeu Amaral Street, Vila Seixas, Ribeirão Preto, São Paulo 14.020-050, Brazil
E-mail addresses: doctor.raulgonzalez@gmail.com; rg@raulgonzalez.com.br

Clin Plastic Surg 41 (2014) 65–72
http://dx.doi.org/10.1016/j.cps.2013.09.015
0094-1298/14/$ – see front matter © 2014 Elsevier Inc. All rights reserved.

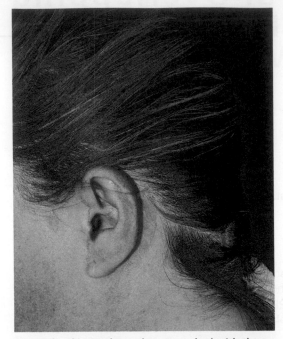

Fig. 1. The skin marks are better marked with the patient awake and standing up. The greater the laxity, the longer the incision. The same holds true with the segment where the incision skirts the hairline before entry into the hairy area.

Undermining and Defatting

The undermining in this procedure is done in two separated parts. The medial third of the face is detached on the areolar plane until 1 cm below the mandibular border, liberating the chin attachments of the skin when necessary. The cervical undermining is done over the platysmal fascia and the fat is left adhered to the skin flap. For didactic purposes, I describe three lines to delimit the borders of the cervical area, which are exposed in this way.[1] The first line marks the posterior border of the platysma muscle, that I call "P"; the second is parallel to the jawline and 1 cm caudal to it; the third, the anterior line, is guided by the second premolar tooth and is called "A." Over this line, the muscle is opened to perform the overlapping plication. All the area included inside the three lines is detached over the platysma fascia. The cervical detachment is done from P to A. On necks with a light degree of laxity, the undermining can stop on line A, but in more severe cases the detachment continues on the same plane to more adequately release the skin to be pulled. The platysma is exposed and I try to leave as much adipose tissue as possible adhered to the skin flap (**Fig. 2**A).

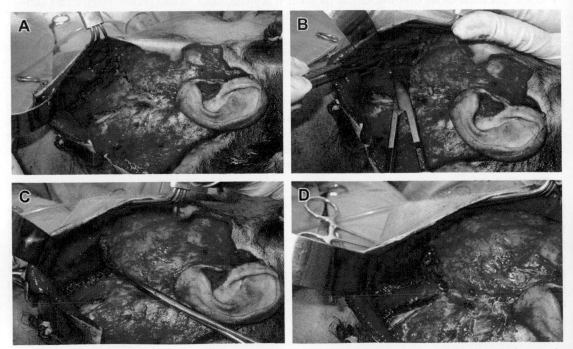

Fig. 2. (*A*) The cervical detachment is always done after the SMAS plication and is undermined entirely over the fascia of the platysma inside the area marked with the three lines: one line over the jawline, another over the posterior edge of the platysma muscle (line P), and one over a line guided by the second premolar tooth. (*B*) Over the line A, the platysma is opened with a pair of scissors and minimally released. (*C*) An Allis forces is pulled strongly up and backward, the anterior edge of the muscular incision, overlapping the muscle over itself. (*D*) The anterior muscular edge is fixed where it arrived with strong absorbable sutures.

The procedures to lift the deep tissue of the midface—*submuscular aponeurotic system* (SMAS) plication, SMAS lifting, or SMASectomies—have to be done before the neck detachment (I usually use a SMASectomy in a majority of cases). When the SMAS is pulled, the fat tissue close to the jaw is pulled together and is raised, changing position. If the SMAS traction is done after cervical undermining, the fat close to the mandible can be positioned too high and create a new jawline higher than desirable. When necessary, an open lipectomy by scissors or liposuction can be done on the skin flap, and, on the medial area, this first defatting is done on the supraplatysma level. The sternocleidomastoideo area can also be defated in order to obtain a thinner neck. This procedure is always done after the work on the SMAS. To better estimate the amount of fat to be resected, I pull up the skin flap to imitate the new neck shape. A suction lipectomy under the platysma on the medial area is easily and safely done through the opening of the muscle on line A.

Tightening the Platysma with an Overlapping Plication

Taking the line A as a guide, I make a vertical incision approximately 3 to 4 cm on the platysma, beginning at 1 cm below the mandibular border and running in the sense of its fibers (see **Fig. 2**B), which creates two edges of muscle, one posterior and one anterior. This line is far from the marginal nerve.[2] This incision gives access to the subplatysmal plane. A small blunt detachment of approximately 1 to 2 cm is required to loosen it and enable traction of the muscular edge thus created (see **Fig. 2**B).

The overlapping maneuver is done using an Allis forceps to pull the anterior edge of the muscle backward and cephalic. Some attempts have to be made, changing the position of the forceps, until the better spot to perform the traction and the fixing suture is determined (see **Fig. 2**C). The anchoring is done by advancing the platysma border by pulling strongly with the forceps and fixating it with a 2-0 Vicryl (Ethicon, Summerville, New Jersey) suture on the platysma, where it arrives, but always right below the mandible, near its angle. The platysma muscle tissue below the mandibular angle is firm and deeply adherent and, therefore, makes for a great anchoring point. The tensile strength adjustment and the tightening of the platysmal tissue right below the mandibular border immediately produce a great definition of the mandibular line (see **Fig. 2**D).

Submandibular Gland Treatment

The submandibular gland (SMG) ptosis, or the gland's caudal displacement, seems to occur due to a slackening of the structures that support the gland caudally, such as the deep fascia of the neck, of which the gland's capsule is an extension, and the platysma muscle.[3] Because of the ptosis, the gland becomes slightly more perceptible, especially in thin people. Some investigators reported their own experience in suspending it or partially removing the gland[3–6] to treat this unaesthetic visibility of the gland; however, they all used a submental incision to approach the gland and they emphasize the complexity of the procedure: little exposure of the surgical field, difficulty to control possible bleeding, and, mainly, the complex anatomy of the area, being close to important vascular and nerve structures. Some experienced surgeons do not advocate a surgical approach to the area due, among other inconveniences, to its complexity and high complication rate.[7]

In my opinion, there are many patients in whom the indication of some treatment to diminish the visibility of gland is unquestionable, but surgeons have been avoiding the procedure due the complexity of performing a partial gland resection. The LOPP method tightens the platysma over the gland and improves subplatysmal structures' support, including the SMG, functioning in a prophylactic way, avoiding the gland bump that may occur after a cervical lift.[1,8–10] At the same time, the LOPP procedure provides safe and easy access to the gland through the muscular incision, thereby making a partial resection of the gland much easier than a complex approach through a submandibular incision.

- With a pair of Allis forceps, the posterior edge of the incision made on the platysma is pulled back, and a small detachment on the subplatysmal tissue easily exposes the gland that sticks out (**Fig. 3**A).
- The gland is infused with Klein solution—the same solution used to infiltrate the face, containing epinephrine. It is strongly advised to wait a few minutes after infusion before cutting in order to obtain a hemostatic effect, because the gland is prone to much bleeding.
- The capsule is opened and an intracapsular dissection is performed.
- Next, the gland is held with a pair of long forceps, leaving out at least 1 cm of the tail, exposing the part to be cut.
- The excision is done with an electric knife, always removing just a little more than 1 cm of the gland's tail (see **Fig. 3**B).

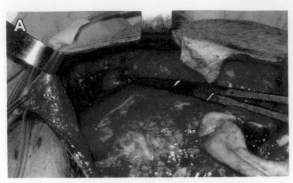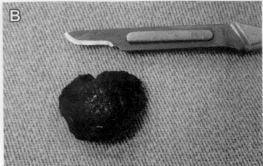

Fig. 3. (A) To expose the SMG, the posterior edge of the muscular opening is pulled posteriorly, and a blunt dissection is done to release the gland of the tissue that covers it. (B) A small portion of the glands tail, a little bit more than 1 cm, is excised using electric knife.

- One or two sutures shaped as an 8 must be done with absorbable suture on the gland's body to stop any possible bleeding and help avoid further bleeding.
- The capsule is also closed with a figure-of-8–shaped raffia suture to embed the gland in its capsule.
- After closing the capsule, the overlapping plication is done on the platysma (see **Fig. 2**C, D).

Digastric Muscle and Other Subplatysmal Structures

In some cases, the tightening obtained by medial plication causes a cephalic displacement of the platysma at the medial line, which is of a different proportion on the lateral area. Because the medial portion rises more than the lateral, where the subplatysmal structures, SMG, and digastric are

located, they become more evident. By tightening the platysma laterally, this finding is noticed less often because the pressure over the subplatysmal structures is closer to these structures than when performed medially.

Platysmal Bands

The platysmal bands are marked with patients awake and standing up and can be treated easily by two methods, the closed platysmotomy, as I describe elsewhere,[1] using strong multibraided threads with needles (**Fig. 4**A,B), and using the platysma incision on line A to cut the marked muscle band with a scissor, making 6 or 7 small horizontal cuts (see **Fig. 4**C–E). These methods have showing effective results on my patients, without recurrence and in light cases can be used as an isolated procedure to treat primary or recurrent bands (see **Fig. 4**F).

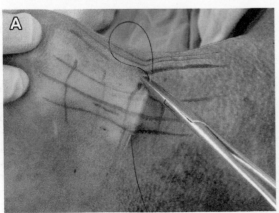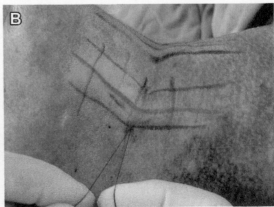

Fig. 4. To perform the closed percutaneous platysmotomy, the skin marks are done with the patient in standing position. The area is well infiltrated and the first incision should be made only after waiting until the hemostatic effect takes place. A 2-0 multibraided nylon with long needle is used to pass the thread first behind the muscle and after, when coming back through the same holes, superficial to it (A). A maneuver with both hands makes a strong back-and-forth movement, like working with a saw, cutting the band on 6 or 7 places (B).

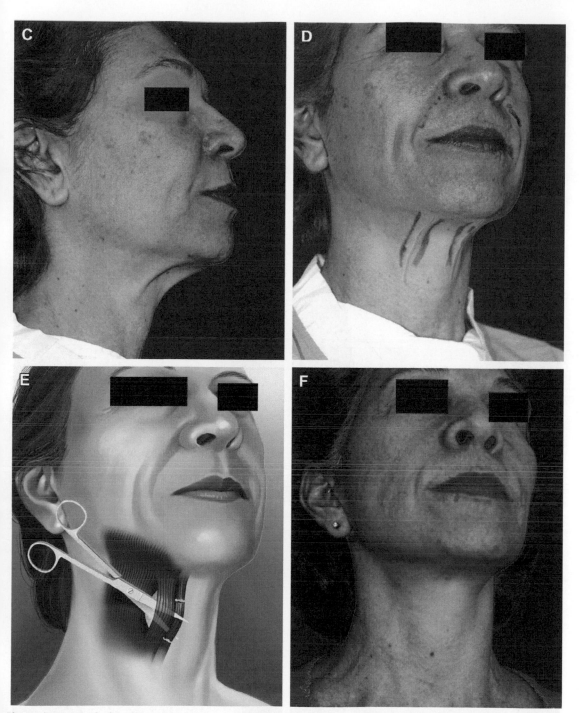

Fig. 4. (*continued*) The platysmal bands are evaluated in rest position (*C*) and marked with the patient standing (*D*). The muscular opening can be used to access the band previously marked and cut with scissors (*E*). Postoperative view of the patient 1 year after the procedure shows no recurrence of the band (*F*).

Medial Plication Versus Lateral Plication

In quantitative terms, the LOPP pull adjusts the platysma in approximately 2.5 cm on each side, totaling 5 cm, whereas by medial plication the adjustment is never higher than 2.5 cm, 3 cm at the most, requiring a surgeon to add other ancillary procedures in some cases, as traction of the lateral edge of the platysma, to achieve more effective tightening. On the other hand, the LOPP is a single procedure providing adequate adjustment of the platysma in all cases. Through the muscular incision, surgeons can expose the SMG, cut platysmal bands, and perform a safe subplatysmal liposuction. This subplatysmal liposuction, when necessary, is done after having performed a superficial liposuction on the supraplatysma level. Using the

muscular opening made on the line A to introduce the cannula, a surgeon is sure that the submandibular nerve is not on the area.

See **Figs. 5** and **6** for clinical view of two patients, preoperative and postoperative LOPP neck lift and additional procedures.

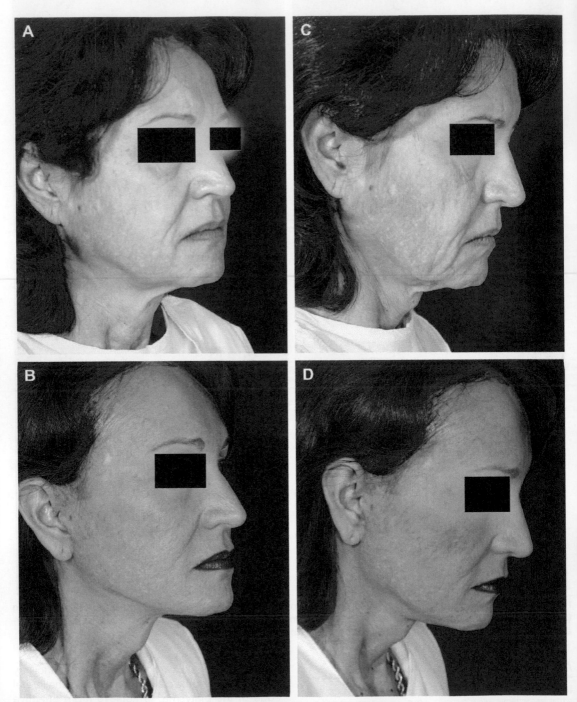

Fig. 5. (*A*) A 56-year-old patient complaining of face and neck laxity. (*B*) Postoperative 11 months after LOPP neck lift and SMASectomy on mid-third of the face. (*C*) Same patient flexing head forward in Connell position. (*D*) Postoperative view.

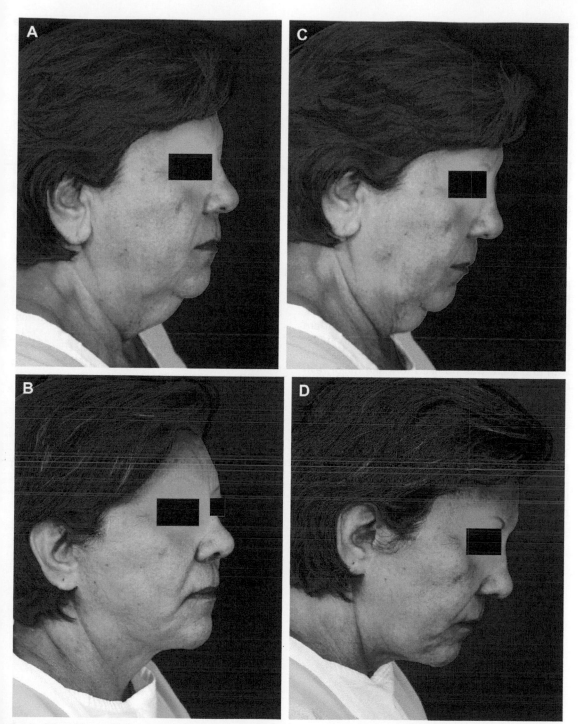

Fig. 6. (*A*) A 67-year-old patient with a heavy neck with very obtuse cervico-mandibular angle. (*B*) Postoperative view 13 months after LOPP neck lift and partial resection of submandibular gland. The anterior belly of the digastric was no touched and the cervical lipectomy was done on subplatysmal level by liposuction and on the skin flap with scissors. (*C*) Same patient flexing head forward in Connell position. (*D*) Postoperative view.

Complications

In my hands, the rate of complications using the LOPP method is much lower than with the former method of medial plication. Necrosis, seromas, irregularities, bumps, and many other problems caused by the large undermining required to perform medial plication are seen less frequently with LOPP. Flap necrosis is one of the most feared complications in facial lifting. It is well known that this problem is closely related to the extension of the undermining and tension of the traction on the flap. With the LOPP procedure, the traction of the muscle flap pulls together the skin, helping to avoid an excessive traction and, because there is a smaller area, undermining the risk of flap necrosis is considerable lower. In addition, the flap is much thicker than that obtained on the areolar plane usually used in medial plications. Although the risk of these complications is small and the rate is lower and, when it happens, is less severe, this method does present complications that are seen on any neck lift; however, in more than 200 cases, all the complications were easy to deal with and there was no need to make major revisions. Any supplementary procedures are done after 6 months.

SUMMARY

The LOOP method can substitute medial plication of the platysma with advantages. It allows surgeons to deal with SMG and platysmal bands in an easier and safer way than when using medial plication. Further experience with this method may lead surgeons to the definitive abandonment of medial plication and its complications.

REFERENCES

1. Gonzalez R. Composite platysmaplasty and closed percutaneous platysma myotomy: a simple way to treat deformities of the neck caused by aging. Aesthet Surg J 2009;29:344.
2. Zairah HA, Atkinson ME. The surgical anatomy of the cervical distribution of the facial nerve. Br J Oral Surg 1981;19(3):171–9.
3. Sullivan PK, Freeman MB, Schmidt S. Contouring the aging neck with submandibular gland suspension. Aesthet Surg J 2006;26:465–71.
4. De Pina DP, Quinta WC. Aesthetic resection of the submandibular salivary gland. Plast Reconstr Surg 1991;88:779–87.
5. Nahai F. The art of aesthetic surgery principles and techniques. Atlanta (Georgia): Quality Medical Publishing; 2005. p. 1239–83.
6. Guyuron B, Jackowe D, Iamphongsai S. Basket submandibular gland suspension. Plast Reconstr Surg 2008 Sep;122(3):938–43.
7. Baker DC. Face lift submandibular gland and digastric muscle resection: radical neck rhytidectomy. Aesthet Surg J 2006;26:85–92.
8. Fogli A. Skin and platysma muscle anchoring. Aesthetic Plast Surg 2008;32:531–41.
9. Labbé D, Franco RG, Nicolas J. Plast Reconstr Surg 2006;117(6):2001–7 [discussion: 2008–10].
10. Feldman JJ. Corset platysmaplasty. Plast Reconstr Surg 1990;85(3):333–43.

Total Neck Rejuvenation Using a Modified Fogli Approach and Selective Resection of Anterior Platysmal Bands

Darryl Hodgkinson, MD, FRCS(C), FACS

KEYWORDS

- Modified Fogli approach • Transverse submental incision • Loré's fascia

KEY POINTS

- Once understood that Loré's fascia was really a thickening of the parotid fascia in the pretragal region and that fascia descended down in front of the facial nerve attaching to the styloid process and the tympanic fissure, it became clear that this skull-based stout ligament had adequate strength to support the traction of the tissues in a permanent way.
- Platysma bands, once resected, do not recur but if observed laterally on animation and found to be disconcerting to the patient, can be treated with botulinum toxin A injections.
- Unfurling of the horizontal wrinkles and the tightening of loose lower neck skin results in a "tallness" of the neck that is best achieved by addressing the entire sternomastoid from the suprasternal region to up behind the angle of the mandible.

 Videos on the author's technique of (1) platysma resection via submental incision; (2) triple cable suture elevating body of platysma; and (3) lower neck tightening with suture fixation platysma to Loré's fascia accompany this article at www.facialplastic.theclinics.com.

Editor Commentary: I have known and I have traded thoughts and concepts with Darryl Hodgkinson for many years. In his chapter, he describes how he has evolved in his management of the platysma muscle including modifying the Fogli technique. Addressing the full vertical height of the platysma muscle as well as correcting horizontal aging changes in the appearance of the neck are important advances in approaching the common problems that often diminish the overall result when not addressed.

INTRODUCTION

Over the past 6 years the author has modified his approach to the aging neck by directing his attention to resecting the redundant platysmal bands after strong superior traction of the body of the platysma muscle to the temporoparotid fascia (Loré's fascia)[1] instead of suturing medial platysmal bands. This technique is a variation of Fogli's initial description,[2] the main difference being that the elevation of the platysma is achieved by a triple cable braided 2/0 suture to the cut edge of Loré's fascia in front of the tragus, affording a strong, permanent elevation of the middle and the lower third of the platysma as well as a horizontal vector. If the horizontal vector is inadequate to improve the jawline in the submental area, a separate submental incision is made to approach the muscles. When this occurs, the redundant muscle bands are resected, not sutured together.

The Cosmetic and Restorative Surgery Clinic, Double Bay Day Surgery, 20 Manning Road, Double Bay, Sydney 2028, Australia
E-mail address: info@cosmeticsurgeryoz.com

Clin Plastic Surg 41 (2014) 73–80
http://dx.doi.org/10.1016/j.cps.2013.09.003
0094-1298/14/$ – see front matter © 2014 Elsevier Inc. All rights reserved.

AESTHETICS AND HISTORY

A tall, well-toned, and distinctly defined neck is synonymous with youth and beauty.[3] Most surgical procedures have focused solely on the upper neck and jaw, improving the definition of the cervicomental angle.

When the author began to perform facelifting procedures in the late 1970s, he was profoundly influenced by Dr Bruce Connell's and others' work[4] in the variety of platysmaplasties that aimed to achieve long-term results in neck rejuvenation. The author used the principles of transection and posterior traction of the platysma for many years. He also incorporated in his technique the work of many authors of the 1980s and 1990s, who manipulated, sutured, transected, and plicated the anterior platysmal bands via the submental incision.[5] The unfortunate recurrence of platysmal bands and associated patient dissatisfaction with the result in the lower neck, especially around the suprasternal notch, was a persistent concern. The author was influenced by Dr Alain Fogli's presentations in 2005 when he published the strong, vertical elevation of the platysma muscle, affixing it to Loré's fascia. The author then began to adopt this maneuver and continued to modify his technique over the subsequent 6 years. His concept has changed to include the rejuvenation of the entire neck from the clavicles to the mastoid region: defining the jawline and the sternomastoid muscle, reducing horizontal wrinkling in the neck, unfurling the neck, and giving the neck the visual appearance of increased height and tone.

Initially Loré's fascia seemed to be an elusive anatomic structure. Once understood, however, that it was really a thickening of the parotid fascia in the pretragal region and that fascia descended down in front of the facial nerve attaching to the styloid process and the tympanic fissure, it was appreciated that this skull-based stout ligament had adequate strength to support the traction of the tissues in a permanent way (**Fig. 1**).[6]

THE ANATOMIC AND FUNCTIONAL PLATYSMA

In 1865, Duchenne demonstrated isolated platysmal contraction by electrophysiological stimulation, which showed that the middle third of the platysma muscle was responsible for horizontal neck wrinkles, shortening, and tightening of the skin across the clavicle as well as a drawing down of the lower lip and mandible.[7]

The trapezoidal-shaped platysma muscles pass obliquely from the mandible, crossing the sternomastoid to insert in the skin of the upper chest.

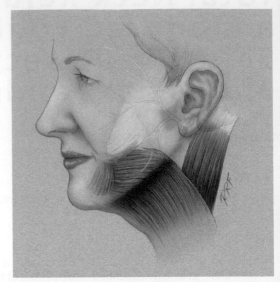

Fig. 1. Loré's tempero parotid fascia in the pretragal area.

Most of the muscles' weight is therefore situated in the lower half of the neck. The 2 plastymal muscles both attach at the mentum, however, with varying degrees of divarication and fascial attachment.[8] As the muscles pass over the mandible, there are fascial attachments of the platysmas to the ramus of the mandible that on contraction lead to an inferior movement of the lower jaw.

The platysma muscles may be quite lax with virtually no motor innervations, dynamic in nature, or spasmodic. Before surgery, the tone in the platysma muscles must be ascertained to determine which bands need to be resected, which bands can be surgically ignored, and which bands can be retracted significantly enough via the described muscle fixation to Loré's fascia.

CLINICAL EVALUATION OF THE PLATYSMA

The patient is asked to contract the platysma muscle by grimacing (**Fig. 2**).

The point where the platsyma crosses the anterior border of the sternomastoid is marked.

The anterior border of the platysma is evaluated for thickness and descent (**Fig. 3**).

If the platysma muscles descend past the thyroid cartilage and are thicker than 1 cm, their planned resection is by submental incision. In a fatty neck, the borders of the platysma are difficult to delineate accurately. A low-lying hyoid and microgenia also impact on the clinical evaluation of an obtuse cervicomental angle. The fat distribution of the neck is either subcutaneous, subplatysmal, or interplatysmal. These fatty deposits, along with the prominence of the submandibular gland and

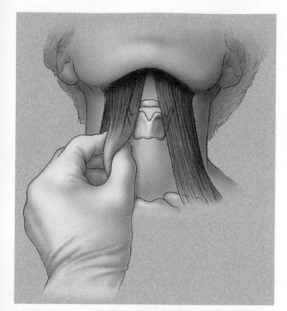

Fig. 2. Preoperative clinical assessment of platysma.

digastric muscles, all impact on the appearance of the aging neck and should be clinically evaluated preoperatively.

PLANNING THE SUBMENTAL INCISION

The submental incision continues to be the most commonly used incision for neck rejuvenation surgery in the over 50-year-old patient. In the author's technique, he assesses which anterior bands are unlikely to be sufficiently elevated by vertical platysmal plication and addresses these via a 4-cm submental incision positioned just anterior to the submental crease (Video 1). The submental incision is also used to insert a chin implant for microgenia or to correct a "witch's chin" deformity.

When the pathologic abnormality of the submental area is difficult to define preoperatively, a "look-see" submental incision is used to identify the subplatysmal and interplatysmal fat pockets as well as the anterior digastric muscle fullness. If thickened digastric muscles are encountered, then these muscles are trimmed to improve the contour of the patient's neck. These heavy muscles are more likely to be encountered in the male patient. The author personally does not resect the submandibular glands but relies on platysmal traction for elevation. The submental area is approached only after the platysma has been elevated and affixed to Loré's fascia on both sides of the neck.

Flaccid anterior plastymal bands, which extend below the apex of the thyroid cartilage and do not contract actively, are ideal for resection. Bands that are more dynamic and extend below the thyroid are more difficult to eliminate with resection and their lateral contraction observed postoperatively can be disconcerting. Regardless, if these bands are prominent, then resection is still required and botulinum toxin A intramuscular injection might be appropriate in these patients if they are still concerned by this lateral animation.

Having resected the bands, the subplatysmal space is entered. If excessive subplastymal or interplatysmal fat is present, it is sharply dissected and judiciously removed. Venous bleeding is regularly encountered during this maneuver. Overresection of these fat pockets is to be avoided because it leads to unwanted "hollowing" in the postoperative appearance. Care must be taken

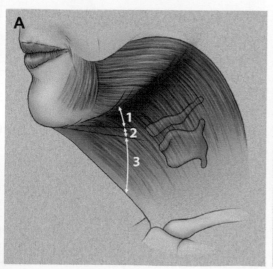

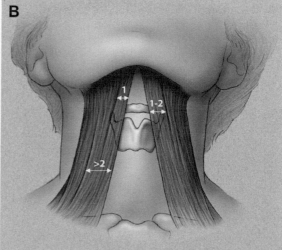

Fig. 3. (*A*) Quantifying descent of platysma below hyoid bone. (*B*) Quantifying the thickness of the platysma bands.

not to thin the anterior skin flap too much because vertical subcutaneous fibrous scar bands can occur and are difficult to manage.

DEFINING THE ANTERIOR STERNOMASTOID MUSCLE

In total neck rejuvenation, the anterior border of the sternomastoid needs to be defined between the mastoid process and the suprasternal notch. A broad strip of the auricular platysmal ligament is incised from the pretragal area down to the platysma, where it obliquely crosses the sternomastoid (**Fig. 4**).

As the triple-cable suture extending from the body of the platysma to Loré's fascia is tied down, it accentuates the anterior border of the sternomastoid by deepening the groove between the angle of the mandible and the muscle (**Fig. 5**, Video 2).

In the inferior dissection, the greater auricular nerve must be avoided, branches of the superior thyroid vessel will be cauterized, and care is taken as the platysma is identified and access is made underneath it to avoid the external jugular vein and its branches (**Fig. 6**).

The position of the suture is predefined at the point where the platysma crosses the anterior border of the sternomastoid. To access this point, the platysma muscle is lifted by forceps, then "scissor spread" underneath the muscle followed by penetration of the muscle and its fascial layers with the needle. To aid in placement of the needle a headlamp and a long bladed lighted retractor are used. The lighted retractor is "towed in" to aid in the elevation of the platysma from its loose underlying fascial attachments. Three passes of the needle between the muscle and the cut edge of Loré's fascia are made.

As the suture is tied down, the skin of the suprasternal notch and lower half of the neck can be observed to tighten (**Fig. 7**, Video 3).

The suture knot is covered by advancement of local submusculo aponeurotic system (S.M.A.S.) at the angle of the mandible or by using the incised

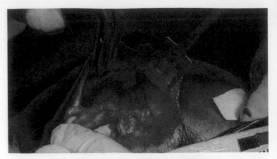

Fig. 5. Triple cable nonabsorbable suture inserted between the cut edge of Loré's fascia and the bulk of the platysma.

flap of platysma auricular ligament, either of which is then sutured back over the knot (**Figs. 8** and **9**).

As the platysma is cinched up, often as much as 3 cm, a significant bulge can occur of excess platysma and S.M.A.S. at the angle of the mandible. The bulge is excised as an S.M.A.S.ectomy similar to Baker's description.[9] The premasseteric space[10] is entered and elevation of the jowl and mid face proceed by figure-of-8 suture fixation with 3/0 absorbable sutures. Skin tethering is inevitable from the considerable elevation of the platysma and S.M.A.S. and requires releasing. Skin redraping and excision are carried out and skin suturing is without tension. Staples are used if a posterior hairline incision is needed. Drains are not used routinely

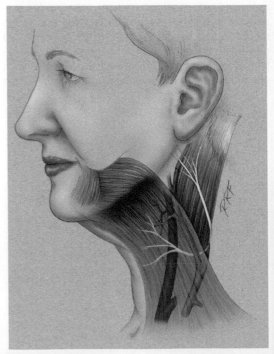

Fig. 6. Anatomic structures to be anticipated in dissection in the taking down of the platysma auricular ligament and suturing of the platysma muscle.

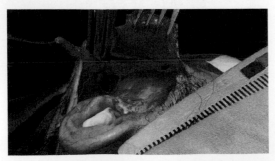

Fig. 4. Platysma auricular ligament incised down to the platysma muscle as it crosses the sternomastoid.

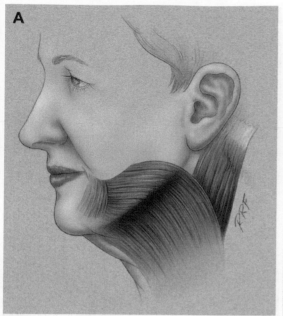
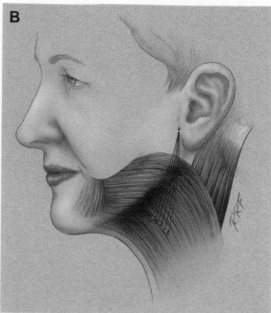

Fig. 7. (*A*) The platysma muscle before elevation. (*B*) Elevation of the body of the platysma and fixation with a triple cable suture to the cut edge of Loré's fascia.

and fibrin glue has never been used. A 1.5-cm gap, which exists without suturing behind the ear, facilitates seroma evacuation. Two-inch paper tape is applied over the areas of dissection. A soft dressing is applied with gauze behind the ears to absorb any seroma. All patients are cared for overnight by the nursing staff, who apply ice continuously and administer prescribed medications for hypertension, nausea, and anxiety as necessary.

RESULTS AND COMPLICATIONS

Table of Complications	
Retrospective Review of 368 Cases 2005–2012	
Hematoma requiring evacuation	6
Seroma requiring aspiration	9
Temporary facial nerve weakness	4
Permanent facial nerve weakness	0
Damage to greater auricular nerve	1
Subcutaneous banding requiring cortisone intralesional injection	3
Return to surgery requiring secondary resection of anterior bands	3
Scar revision including correction of pixie ear deformity	4
Dissatisfaction at 6 mo	2
Secondary lift in less than 2 y for persistent or recurrent laxity	3

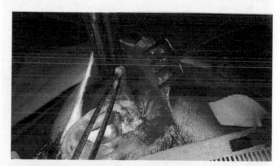

Fig. 8. Resected platysma auricular ligament elevated and sutured over triple cable suture.

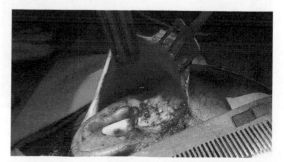

Fig. 9. Resected auricular ligament reattached to the cut edge of Loré's fascia over the triple cable nonabsorbable suture.

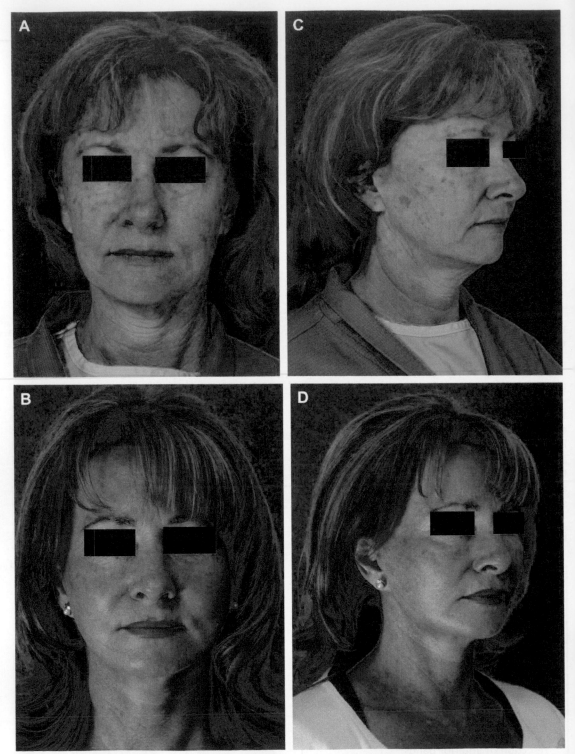

Fig. 10. Frontal view of a 59-year-old patient before (*A*) and after (*B*) facelift using Loré's fascia fixation of platysma. Oblique view of a 59-year-old patient before (*C*) and after (*D*) facelift using Loré's fascia fixation of platysma.

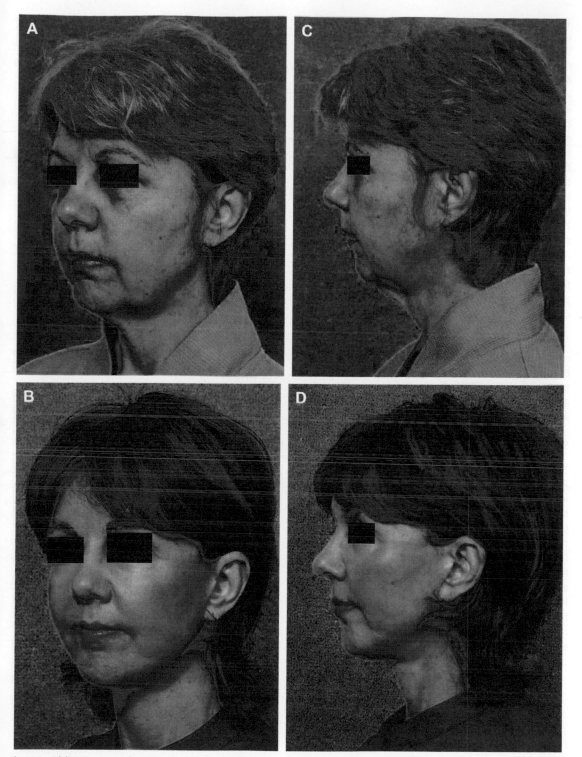

Fig. 11. Oblique view of a 51-year-old patient before (*A*) and after (*B*) upper and lower lid blepharoplasty and facelift using Loré's fascia fixation of platysma. Lateral view of a 51-year-old patient before (*C*) and after (*D*) upper and lower lid blepharoplasty and facelift using Loré's fascia fixation of platysma.

This is not a limited incision or limited dissection procedure except in the younger, fatty-necked patients where liposuction is the main component of neck sculpting. The hematoma rate in greater than 400 cases is less than 2% and is not correlated with the submental incisional approach. Specifically related to this technique have been 2 cases of infection around the braided suture, requiring suture knot removal. In a very few patients the suture has been palpable, which further emphasizes the need to cover the heavy knot fully with local tissue advancement especially in the thin patient.

In the 1-year postoperative follow-up of patients, some laxity of the skin under the chin has been noted, particularly in patients who have had excessive exposure to the sun, as is common in Australia. Platysma bands once resected do not recur but if observed laterally on animation and found to be disconcerting to the patient, can be treated with botulinum toxin A injections as previously mentioned.

Most gratifying is the unfurling of the horizontal wrinkles and the tightening of loose lower neck skin, resulting in a "tallness" of the neck, which is best achieved by addressing the entire sternomastoid from the suprasternal region to up behind the angle of the mandible. **Figs. 10** and **11** demonstrate the clinical results.

SUMMARY

This approach to neck rejuvenation over the past 7 years has applied Dr Alain Fogli's[11] principle of vertical platysma fixation to Loré's fascia. The author's variation involves a transverse incision in Loré's fascia in the pretragal region, a "takedown" of the auriculoplatysmal ligament by resection to the body of the platysma where it crosses the sternomastoid muscle and then a triple cable suture fixation to the cut edge of Loré's fascia. Platysma bands are assessed for their degree of redundancy and those judged excessive in thickness or descent are resected via a submental incision. The subsequent strong fixation with the triple cable braided suture tightens the lower half of the platysma and defines the lower half of the sternomastoid muscle.

More extensive surgery is appropriate when and if a superior result can be achieved, such as the creation of a tall, tight neck, a feature that is synonymous with female youth and beauty.

SUPPLEMENTARY DATA

Supplementary data related to this article can be found at http://dx.doi.org/10.1016/j.cps.2013.09.003.

REFERENCES

1. Hodgkinson DJ. Five-year experience with modified Fogli (Loré's fascia fixation) platysmaplasty (2012). Aesthetic Plast Surg 2012;36:28–40.
2. Fogli AL. Skin and platysma muscle anchoring. Aesthetic Plast Surg 2008;32:531–41.
3. Ellenbogen R, Karlin JV. Visual criteria for success in youthful neck. Plast Reconstr Surg 1980;66:826–37.
4. Connell BF. Contouring the neck in rhytidectomy by lipectomy and muscle sling. Plast Reconstr Surg 1978;61:376–83.
5. Fuente del Campo A. Facial aesthetic surgery: the hammock platysmaplasty. Aesthet Surg J 1998;18:246–52.
6. Loré JM. An atlas of head and neck surgery, vol. 2. Philadelphia: W.B. Saunders; 1973. p. 596.
7. Duchenne de Boulogne B. The mechanism of human facial expression. Cambridge: Cambridge University Press; 1990. p. 89–92.
8. De Castro C. The anatomy of the platysma muscle. Plast Reconstr Surg 1980;66:680–7.
9. Baker DC. Lateral SMASectomy plication and short scar facelifts: indications and techniques. Clin Plast Surg 2008;35:533–50.
10. Mendelson BC, Freeman ME, Wu W, et al. Surgical anatomy of the lower face: the pre-masseter space, the jowl and the labiomandibular fold. Aesthetic Plast Surg 2008;32:185–95.
11. Fogli AL, Desouches C. Less invasive facelifting. Clin Plast Surg 2008;35:519–29.

Neck Contouring

Patrick Trevidic, MD

KEYWORDS

- Neck lift • Plastic surgery • Neck contouring • Surgical complications • Surgical technique
- Platysma • Submaxillary • Jowls

KEY POINTS

- Maximum defating of the jowl and the neck.
- Minimum defating of the middle third.
- Anterior neck dissection only for difficult case.
- Botulinum toxin for submaxillary gland and early platysma bands recurrence.

Editor Commentary: I met Patrick when he kindly asked me to participate in a anatomy laboratory teaching session in Paris. We have remained close friends and I have learned a lot from him. In addition to this contribution, his books on the anatomy of Botulinun toxin injetions and facial fillers provide safe, sound methods to chemically rejuvenate the face and neck. His treatment of the submaxillary glands and recurrent platysma bands with Botulinum Toxin, included in this chapter is important to have in our list of procedures.

INCISION

Typically, for the young female patient with a thin neck, I use only the classical skin incision of face lifting, with no anterior approach.

For the older male patient with a heavy neck, platysma bands and retrogenia, I begin with an anterior approach and I add a classical face lifting incision.

I never use only an anterior approach in a patient who is undergoing facelift for the first-time, but I sometimes do in cases of recurrence of neck ptosis following a first facelift.

DEFAT AND FAT GRAFTING

To defat the neck I use only liposuction, but extensively, systematically including the jowl above the platysma and between the anterior platysma's bands, ceasing the liposuction at the mandibular line.

I leave skin only with no fat above the neck platysma. This is done to reinforce the angle between the mandibular line (where I keep the fat) and the neck (where there is no more fat above the platysma).

I do not perform a fat resection because, between the anterior bellies of the digastric muscle, it is impossible to avoid the lymphatic nodes and vessels located in the sub mental area. Moreover, fat resection can create irregularity, asymmetry, bumps and hardness in the area, making patient follow up and recurring visits challenging.

MUSCLES

I never resect the anterior bellies of the digastric muscle in order to avoid skinny neck and "widow like" or "witch's" chin.

When I have completed the liposuction, by my anterior approach, I undermine the anterior border of the platysma and I perform a corset platysmarraphy with a barbed suture (like QUILL®) up to the superior border of the thyroid cartilage **(Fig. 1)**.

Scientific Director, Expert2expert group, Paris, France
E-mail address: patrick.trevidic@orange.fr

Clin Plastic Surg 41 (2014) 81–83
http://dx.doi.org/10.1016/j.cps.2013.10.001
0094-1298/14/$ – see front matter © 2014 Elsevier Inc. All rights reserved.

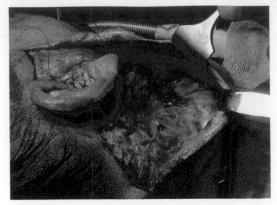

Fig. 1. Skin undermining following total neck lipoaspiration.

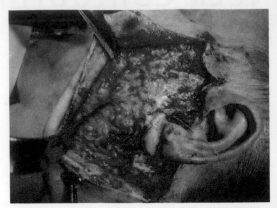

Fig. 2. Anchoring points between the skin and the tightened SMAS.

The back cut is only done by the classical face lifting approach when I suture with a vertical vector the platysma on the LORE's fascia.

SUBMAXILLARY GLAND

A visible sub maxillary gland can be spontaneous or can occur after a liposuction combined or not with a facelift.

In cases of appearance of sub maxillary gland, I use Botulinum toxin inside the gland (50 Speywood units or 20 international units per side), two or three treatments with an interval of 4 months between each treatment.

SKIN

The main point is how to pull on the skin with an anterior or lateral approach because the action

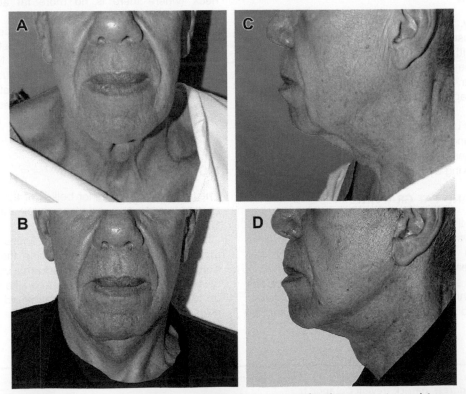

Fig. 3. Outcome after 1 year showing a fast recurrence of neck ptosis. (*A–B*) Preoperative and 1-year postoperative front views. (*C–D*) Preoperative and 1 year postoperative side views.

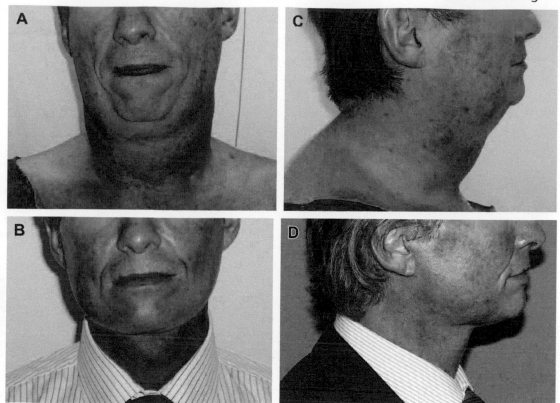

Fig. 4. Good outcome after 2 years.

on the skin is never complete due to the fact that the site of action is too far to reach even through an SMAS lifting.

Therefore, the idea, after you have tightened the deep plane, is to create a high anterior tension with anchoring points - 4 to 5 side by side - linking the dermis to the deep plane (**Fig. 2**).

These points disappear after few weeks and will avoid the occurrence of a dead space anteriorly.

DRAINS

I drain the inferior part of my neck by my classical face lifting approach.

COMPLICATION

The main early complication is hematoma, as with every face lifting, and mainly with the male patient with high blood pressure medical condition.

To avoid hematoma I use a continuous blood pressure follow up protocol during 12 hours, with Loxen® injection if pressure is above 120 mm Hg.

The main late complication with the neck lift technique is to have hypo correction or a fast recurrence. If recurrence is on the platysma bands, I start correcting that with botulinum toxin injection (40 Speywood side by side) or, if it doesn't work, I do an anterior approach alone.

Fig. 3 shows a recurrence of neck ptosis. **Fig. 4** shows good outcome neck lift 1 year postoperative.

SUGGESTED READINGS

Jones BM, Lo SJ. How long does a face lift last? Objective and subjective measurements over a 5-year period. Plast Reconstr Surg 2012;130(6):1317–27. http://dx.doi.org/10.1097/PRS.0b013e31826d9f7f.

Jones BM, Grover R. Avoiding hematoma in cervicofacial rhytidectomy: a personal 8-year quest. Reviewing 910 patients. Plast Reconstr Surg 2004;113(1): 381–7 [discussion: 388–90].

Lindsey WH, Zapanta PE. Direct excision of the turkey jowl deformity: a review of 100 consecutive cases. Arch Facial Plast Surg 2007;9(1):56–61.

Matarasso A, Elkwood A, Rankin M, et al. National plastic surgery survey: face lift techniques and complications. Plast Reconstr Surg 2000;106(5):1185–95 [discussion: 1196].

Marten TJ, Feldman JJ, Connell BF, et al. Treatment of the full obtuse neck. Aesthet Surg J 2005; 25(4):387–97. http://dx.doi.org/10.1016/j.asj.2005. 04.005.

Pitanguy I, Machado BH. Facial rejuvenation surgery: a retrospective study of 8788 cases. Aesthet Surg J 2012;32(4):393–412. http://dx.doi.org/10. 1177/1090820X12438895.

Managing the Components of the Aging Neck
From Liposuction to Submentalplasty, to Neck Lift

Alan Matarasso, MD

KEYWORDS

- Aging neck • Management • Neck lift • Liposuction • Submentalplasty

KEY POINTS

- The neck can be treated independently from the face.
- Procedures range from liposuction to Submentalplasty, to a necklift.
- The neck lift can be extended to include treatment of the jowls.

Editor Commentary: Alan begins with several quotes that tell denote the importance of the aging neck. He takes us through his algorhythm which may include panfacial rejuvenation based upon the clinical findings. He is willing to perform isolated neck rejuvenation as indicated, but frequently more is required. He also will approach the subject of ancillary procedures such as chin augmentation and partial resection of the submaxillary glands which can have a subtle yet important effect on the final result. This approach cleverly allows the patient to guide the surgeon after being armed with the pertinent information.

INTRODUCTION/OVERVIEW

"I often do what so many women my age do when in front of a mirror: I gently pull the skin of my neck back and stare wistfully at a younger version of myself."

"Oh, the necks. There are chicken necks. There are turkey gobbler necks. There are elephant necks. There are necks with waddles and necks with creases that are on the verge of becoming waddles. There are scrawny necks, wrinkled necks, mottled necks. There are necks that are an amazing combination of all of the above. According to my dermatologist, the neck starts at forty-three and that's that."

"You can put makeup on your face and concealer under your eyes and dye on your hair, you can shoot collagen and Botulinum Toxin and fillers into your wrinkles and creases, but short of surgery, there's not a damn thing you can do about a neck. The neck is a dead giveaway. Our faces are lies and our necks are the truth."

"This is about my neck. And I know what you are thinking: Why not go to a plastic surgeon? I'll tell you why not. If you go to a plastic surgeon and say, I'd like you just to fix my neck, he will tell you flat out that he can't do it without giving you a face-lift too. And he's not lying. He's not trying to con you into spending more money, The fact is, it's all one big ball of wax. If you tighten up the neck, you've also got to tighten up the face."[1]

The neck, the region from the jawline to the collarbone and, to some degree, the jowls or what patients may refer to as their chin, is

Plastic Surgery, Manhattan Eye, Ear & Throat Hospital, Lenox Hill Hospital, North Shore-Long Island Jewish Health System, 1009 Park Avenue, New York, NY 10028, USA
E-mail address: dam@drmatarasso.com

Clin Plastic Surg 41 (2014) 85–98
http://dx.doi.org/10.1016/j.cps.2013.09.013
0094-1298/14/$ – see front matter © 2014 Elsevier Inc. All rights reserved.

undeniably a common concern for patients. The aforementioned quotes by bestselling author Nora Ephron accurately depict the following about the neck: (1) From the late 30s onward, people invariably pull up on the excess skin, attempting to picture a less-aged version of themselves. (2) It is a telltale, inevitable sign of aging. (3) Unlike the face, there are limited nonsurgical treatments that are beneficial. However, in contrast to Ephron's last quote, the neck can be isolated from the face and treated independently. This article focuses on the surgical management of the aging neck.

Ellenbogen[2] has described the ideal appearance of a youthful neck. With advancing age, these features inevitably change. Several factors contribute to the senescence of the neck, which have to be analyzed and potentially addressed, including the quality and the quantity of the skin, the subcutaneous and subplatysmal adipose tissue, the status of the platysma muscle (and possibly the digestive muscles), the bony architecture of the mandible, and the submandibular glands. The skin quality is particularly important because no amount of pulling, despite what patients may think, will improve damaged skin. Indeed the swelling of surgery often makes damaged skin look temporarily improved; as that wanes, patients want more surgical tightening in a vain attempt to improve what is actually damaged skin. Furthermore, the relationship with neck aging to the jowls/jawline and the midface should be evaluated, including how full the midface is. **Box 1** describes regions related that may or may not be concomitantly addressed at the time of neck surgery.

The consultation begins with a clear understanding of the patients' concerns (eg, their goals, their dislikes, their tolerance for incisions, how long a recovery period they are willing to accept, and so forth) and reconciling their issues with the surgeon's physical findings and their anatomy. Periodically, it is prudent to appropriately suggest concomitant related procedures, such as chin enhancement,[3] buccal fat pad removal,[4] or reduction in the salivary gland size, all of which can have a direct impact on the appearance of the neck after surgery. Naturally, the traditional concept of a facelift, which includes the area from cheek to collarbone, is a frequent component of the discussion. With regard to the midface area, patients can be under the misconception that it is necessary to include the midface in the surgical procedure for a neck lift or they may prefer nonsurgical methods (lasers, neurotoxins, or fillers) to improve the face itself. However, for neck laxity, surgical rejuvenation is the only reliable option. In the author's experience, patients are interested in neck surgery alone because (1) that is all that concerns them, (2) their midface is adequately addressed with nonsurgical treatments, or (3) they prefer not to have the preauricular scar associated with facelift surgery. It is quite clear physiologically and in the judgment of patients that the neck ages differently than the face. Whether or not patients have had facial rejuvenation surgery previously, the neck is usually a significant appearance concern. Consequently, the ability to isolate and surgically treat the neck alone is now an increasingly popular option for patients seeking surgical intervention.

Patients often want to have a preview of the surgical outcome. To experience this, they commonly pull back neck tissue manually in opposing directions with their fingers (the "finger-pull" test). Although helpful in certain circumstances, this can also be misleading, especially if surgery does not entirely eliminate the platysma bands despite how it appears when pulling back on the skin. A more realistic preview may be achieved by looking at themselves in a mirror while lying on their back.

PREOPERATIVE PLANNING

Preoperative planning is ultimately a matter of reconciling the patients' goals with their anatomy. The author explains to patients what their physical findings are and advise them of the role of surgery (addressing skin, fat, and muscle in the neck), the role of nonsurgical procedures (addressing the quality of the skin itself), and the value of topical products. Then the author creates and explains an algorithm to them (**Table 1**) based on the treatable components of the aging neck and discusses

---

Box 1
Related components to correct neck aging

- Submandibular glands
- Jowls
- Marionette lines
- Hypertrophic earlobes
- Microgenia
- Buccal lipodystrophy
- Larynx[a]
- Masseter muscle hypertrophy
- Parotid gland enlargement

[a] Potentially addressed in conjunction with neck surgery.

Table 1
Decision analysis and patient education in treating soft tissue components in the aging neck

Fat	*Muscle	Skin	Treatment
+	No laxity	Adequate	Liposuction
+	+	Adequate	Submentalplasty
+/−	+	+	Neck lift[a]

* Visible or lax medial border platysma bands (submentalplasty) muscle treatments include resection, plication (Eiffel Tower), or incising.

These components (skin, fat, muscle) represent a framework for analyzing a range of neck deformities.

[a] Within neck lift, it often includes submentalplasty.

the impact that surgery can be expected to have. The algorithm is essentially that patients with a younger, fattier neck are treated with liposuction (**Fig. 1**), patients with an early aging neck are treated with a submentalplasty (**Fig. 2**) (submental incision, liposuction, platysma surgery, and no skin excision), and more advanced patients are treated with a neck lift (liposuction, submentalplasty, and then flap elevation and skin excision) (**Figs. 3** and **4**). Essentially, each of the 3 common surgical alternatives is cumulative, with each incorporating the earlier technique as they advance from liposuction to a submentalplasty and finally to a neck lift. Despite that algorithm, patients may prefer to downstage their choice of operation to less-invasive options because of a variety of personal concerns. But they should be firmly aware that less-invasive procedures do not yield the same result, understanding that a downstaged, less-invasive procedure can achieve a suitable, albeit less complete, outcome if it coincides with their goals (**Figs. 5** and **6**).

The neck lifts that the author performs include a traditional one (**Fig. 7**), which addresses the area from the jawline down, or an extended neck lift (**Fig. 8**), which, in addition to the aforementioned area, also improves the jowl area because the incision advances cephalically for a short distance preauricularly, which allows for additional jowl skin tightening and lower sub muscular aponeurotic system (SMAS) advancement. Jowl liposuction frequently accompanies either variation of a neck lift.

OPERATIVE TECHNIQUE

The neck lift is performed in an accredited ambulatory facility under systemic anesthesia administered by an anesthesiologist.

- The field is injected with a wetting solution containing 1 mL of 1:1000 epinephrine, 100 mL of 1% lidocaine, and 200 mL of normal saline.
- Neck lift surgery begins with liposuction of the subcutaneous fat as indicated.
- A 2.4-mm Mercedes cannula is used for neck liposuction and 1.8-mm Mercedes cannula used for liposuction of the jowl area.
- In closed procedures (Suction assisted lipectomy [SAL] alone) or very fatty necks, additional liposuction is performed with a spatula tip cannula.
- A submental incision is made just above or below the natural submental crease when midline platysma muscle (**Fig. 9**A) access is necessary.
- Wide undermining of the neck is performed with the aid of a lighted fiber-optic retractor and countertraction on the skin. Medial platysma bands are then identified. Various configurations of the midline platysma muscle repair have been described.[5,6]
- In those patients with loose redundant or hypertrophic anterior platysma bands, the author begins by excising a strip of excess platysma muscle (see **Fig. 9**B). Submuscular fat can then be identified. If patients will benefit by reducing it, the author gently teases and excises a small amount out and melts some by coagulation with a ball-tip electrocautery.
- Attention is then returned to the platysma muscle, which is first back cut at the level of the hyoid bone. Depending on the integrity of the muscle, it is either repaired in the midline in layers with a 3-0 mersilene (Ethicon, San Lorenzo, Puerto Rico) sutures which, when complete, resembles an Eiffel Tower. Alternatively, the platysma can be serially interrupted at regular intervals by cutting through the muscle with a Colorado needle (Stryker, Kalamazoo, MI) and electrocautery.
- With the patients' head turned, surgery continues on the right side of the neck where the incisions are demarcated.
- The skin flaps are incised sharply and undermined under direct vision with a knife and facelift scissors. Most of the time, the neck is undermined completely from side to side, joining where the submental dissection began earlier. The lower border of the SMAS (in extended neck lifts) is identified, and the lateral border of the platysma is located and evaluated.
- In situations where the platysma is lax or redundant, it is undermined and sutured to the sternocleidomastoid (SCM) fascia without

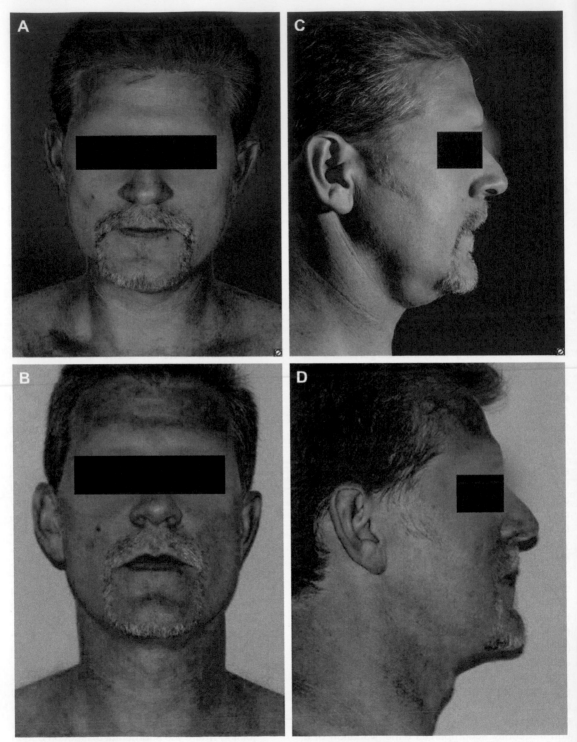

Fig. 1. Younger, fattier neck treated with liposuction. (*A*) Pre procedural front view. (*B*) Post liposuction front view. (*C*) Pre procedural right profile view. (*D*) Post liposuction right profile view.

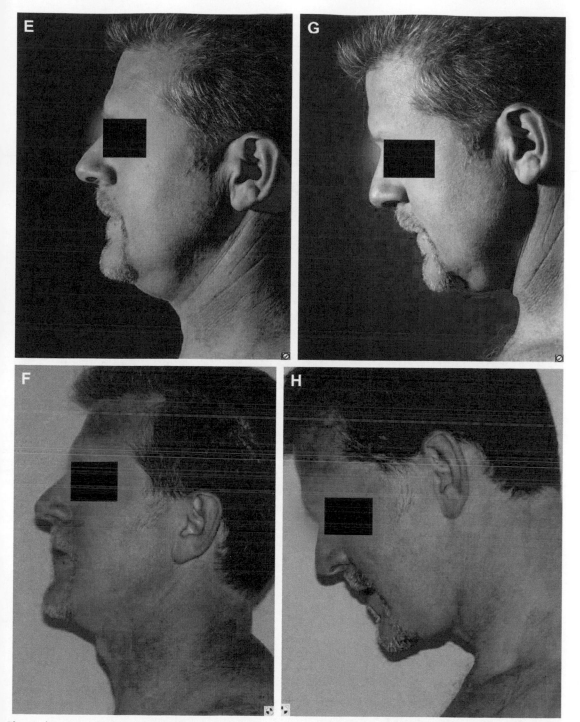

Fig. 1. (*continued*) (*E*) Pre procedural left profile view. (*F*) Post liposuction left profile view. (*G*) Pre procedural, patient with head leaning down. (*H*) Post liposuction, head leaning down.

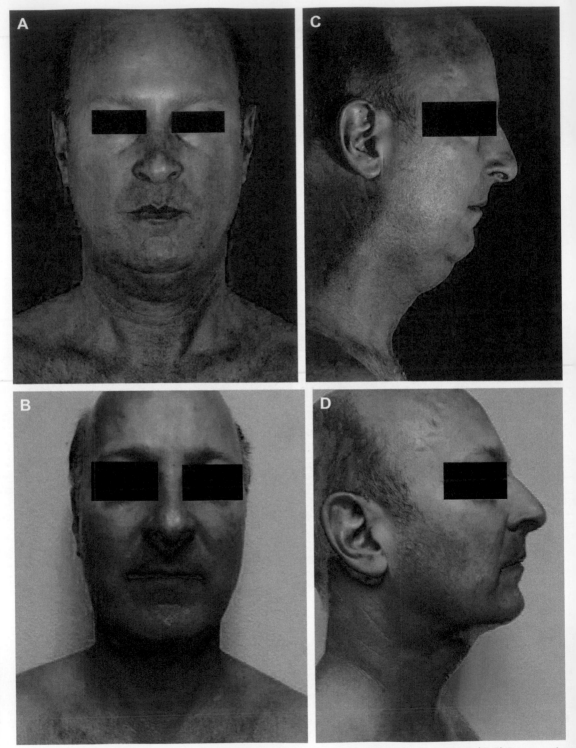

Fig. 2. Submentalplasty, BFP, BL2 UL. (*A, B*) Preoperative and 1-year postoperative front view. (*C, D*) Preoperative and 1-year postoperative lateral view. BFP, buccal fat pad; BL2 UL, upper lid blepharoplasty.

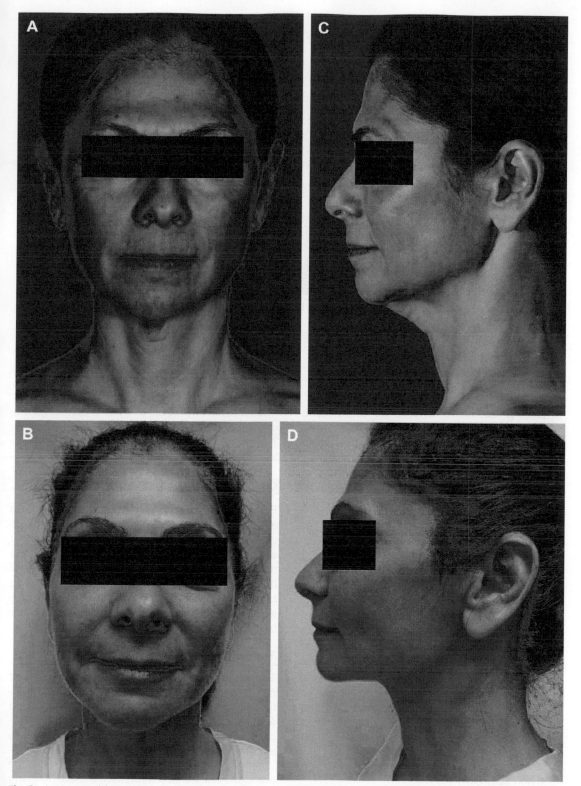

Fig. 3. A 54-year old woman concerned with neck laxity. (*A–D*) Front and lateral views before and after a neck lift.

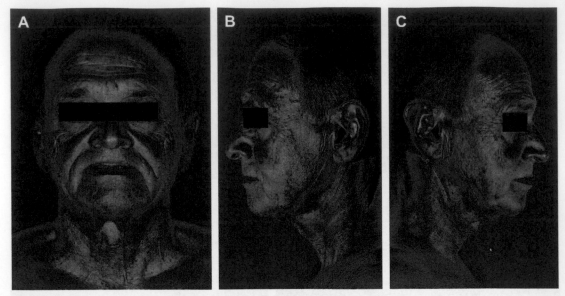

Fig. 4. A 66-year-old man with an aging neck. (*A–C*) Before and after neck lift.

placing excessive tension on the midline repair.

- In other cases, the platysma is plicated to the SCM at 3 points with a 3-0 mersilene suture, including the lower SMAS for jowl improvement.
- Final hemostasis is achieved by electrocautery.
- In facelift surgery, the author prefers to spray a fibrin sealant and not use drains because, with the short scar facelift, the drains exacerbate the inevitable skin pleating that occurs postauricularly.
- In contrast, in a neck lift, skin bunching (pleating) does not occur, so drains are used, brought out through the wound, and secured with an absorbable suture.
- Excess skin is elevated, advanced, redraped, and excised so as to optimize the result and preserve the integrity of the hairline. The hair-bearing area is closed with staples, and the bridge between the hair-bearing skin and postauricular incision is closed with half-buried absorbable sutures.
- The postauricular crease is closed with 3-0 nylon sutures.
- Antibiotic ointment is applied to all wounds.
- A standard 2-layer facelift dressing consisting of gauze and surginet (Dermapac, Shelton, CT) is placed on the patients.

Noticeable hypertrophic submandibular glands can be treated with botulinum toxin injections. The author does not routinely resect submandibular glands or digastric muscles.

COMPLICATIONS

Patients frequently inquire about the need for chin augmentation. The author explains the parameters used to determine the indications for surgery and suggests that the chin looks better once the neck is improved. A reliable way to help patients decide is for them to recall if their chin always bothered them. If it did not, the neck surgery alone is frequently sufficient. If it did previously bother them, chin augmentation is then discussed.

Scarring and Hematoma in Neck Lift

The apex of the postauricular incision is most prone to ischemia or hypertrophic scarring; therefore, tension on wound closure should be adjusted accordingly, and patients should avoid hyperflexing the neck in the early postoperative period to ensure adequate vascularization.

Small, nonexpanding hematomas can be managed in a sterile environment without returning to the operating room. Blood is suctioned out from under the flap, and then the wound is irrigated with a solution containing cold saline mixed with local anesthesia and epinephrine. Gentle pressure is

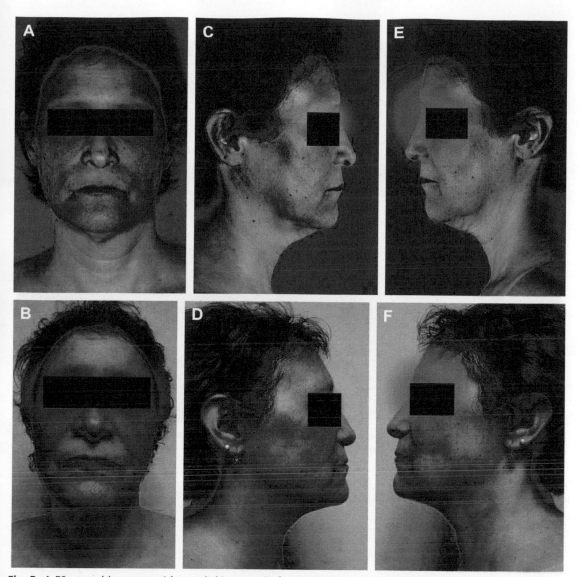

Fig. 5. A 59-year old woman with good skin tone. Before and after neck liposuction alone. She also had a 4-lid blepharoplasty and large-volume liposuction of abdomen and flanks. A, C, and E show the patient pre procedure. B, D, and F show the patient post procedure.

applied; this sequence continues until the output appears clearer.

Larger or expanding hematomas should be treated emergently in an operating room. The affected area is completely exposed, inspected, treated, and the wound drained. When indicated, a workup for bleeding disorders should be considered.

Deep Vein Thrombophlebitis or Pulmonary Embolism in Neck Lift

Deep vein thrombophlebitis (DVT) and pulmonary embolism (PE) are rare events in neck lift surgery. Preoperative precautions, such as ceasing

nicotine use and hormones, are recommended. A history of excessive bleeding or miscarriages, which can be a marker for prothrombotic factors, should be addressed. Precautions, including TED stockings/sequential pneumatic compression devices, are routinely used. If a DVT/PE is suspected based on the history and physical findings D-dimers and spiral computed tomography scans are useful in the diagnosis. Prompt therapy despite it being during the postoperative period should be initiated. At some point, special hematology (hypercoagulation workup) can be obtained to investigate genetic prothrombotic disorders that lend themselves to a propensity toward blood clotting.

A

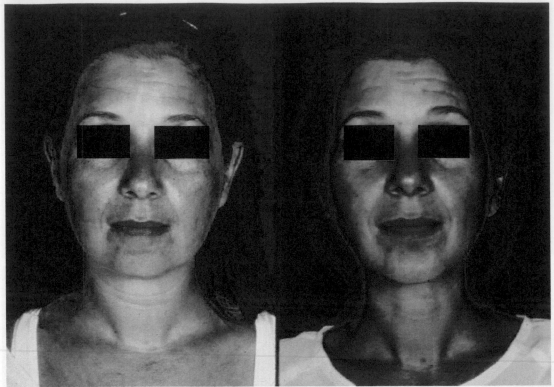

Fig. 6. Patient requesting a minimally invasive alternative. Before (*A*) and after (*B*) liposuction of the neck, excision of buccal fat pads, and Silastic (Dow Corning Corporation, Midland, MI) chin implants.

Seromas in Neck Lift

Seromas can occur in neck lift surgery. A balatable fluid wave should prompt a high degree of suspicion for the presence of fluid. These seromas should be aspirated and the area compressed (eg, elastic head strap). Patients should be examined frequently because there is a tendency for these to reoccur. Seromas need to be aggressively treated in order to ensure complete evacuation of the fluid. Persistent or recurrent fluid that is not evacuated results in a long-term contour defect not readily amenable to any intervention, particularly in the midline. These contour deformities tend to resolve gradually over a period of time during which time they appear as an unsightly contour abnormality (**Fig. 10**).

Infections in Neck Lift

Wound infections are also infrequent but should be promptly recognized and appropriately treated

with antibiotics. Left untreated, they can lead to a cascade of complications, including extensive tissue ischemia.

Skin Ischemia in Neck Lift

Skin ischemia should be evaluated for reversible causes, such as fluid collections, infections, extensive skin tension, and so forth; if identified, they are treated. Should ischemia progress to necrosis, it should be managed with observation and local wound care until final demarcation. Areas of suspected ischemia may be improved with RMSO/DMSO (Spectrum Chemical MFG Corp, Gardena, CA). Once frank necrosis is apparent, wounds can be treated with silver sulfadiazine (Silvadene) cream. Bovey burns of the skin flap can also occur; these tend to be larger than anticipated and are invariably full thickness. They can be managed similarly to skin flap ischemia and

B

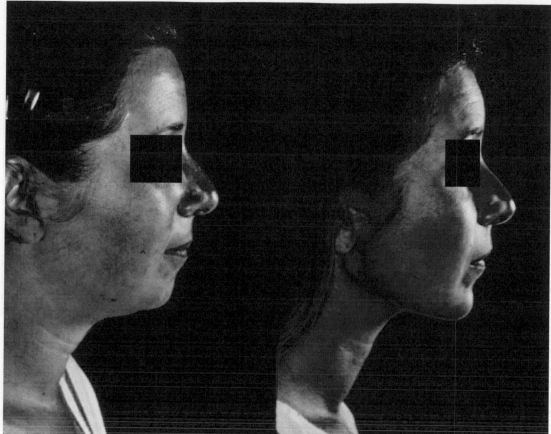

Fig. 6.

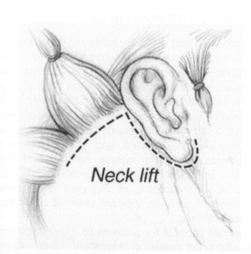

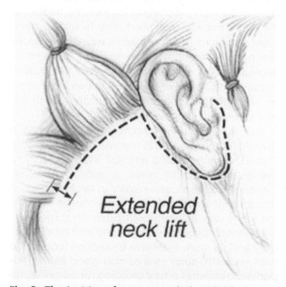

Fig. 7. The incisions for a neck lift.

Fig. 8. The incisions for an extended neck lift.

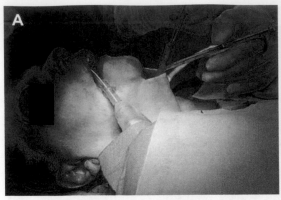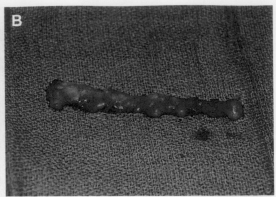

Fig. 9. (*A*) Submental incision that provides access to the midline platysma. (*B*) Wedge medial platysma muscle excised during a neck lift.

necrosis. The author occasionally also uses beca-plermin (Regranex) on these sites.

Facial Nerve Injury in Neck Lift

Facial nerve injuries are less common in neck lifts than in facelifts in the author's experience. The marginal mandibular is at risk of injury from lipo-suction in the jowl area or from subplatysmal sur-gery in the neck. The cervical branch is at risk from midline platysma surgery. In scenarios of secondary neck surgery accompanied by sub-mentalplasty, the cervical branch is most suscep-tible to injury. Consequently, care must be given before considering secondary midline platysma surgery. Injury to that nerve results in a psuedo-marginal mandibular injury appearance.[7,8] These potentially highly disturbing injuries are treated in the same manner described after facelift surgery. Most situations of nerve injuries will resolve spon-taneously over time within the first 6 months, although some can take up to 1 year. Gradual or partial appearance of muscle function innervated by an injured nerve correlates positively with the ultimate return of nerve function.

The skin is routinely numb feeling following a neck lift surgery, and this resolves spontaneously. This event is expected and self-limiting. Injury to the greater auricular nerve, a sensory nerve, is the most common nerve injury in neck surgery. It occurs in the same manner and can be avoided the same way as one would in facelift surgery.

Other complications associated with facelift sur-gery and its more extensive dissection (compared with neck lift), such as a parotid gland fistula, su-perficial temporal artery bleeding, or alopecia, do not occur in neck surgery.

Recurrent Platysma Bands After Neck Lift

Persistent or recurrent platysma bands despite appropriate treatment are reported and probably occur more commonly than anticipated. This can be caused by the more lateral aspects of the mus-cle accordion inward and overlapping. I explain this to patients as the platysma muscle being anal-ogous to the curtain of a movie theater. When the central gap of the curtain (medial border of the pla-tysma muscle) is closed, adjacent lateral pleats in the curtain can prolapse medially; therefore creating recurrent platysma bands. They can be managed with botulinum toxin injections or reop-erated on. Bowstringing of surgically repaired midline platysma bands can be reduced by inter-rupting the band and excising a triangular wedge at the base of the platysma muscle where the su-ture repair begins.

POSTOPERATIVE MANAGEMENT

The dressing and drain are removed on postoper-ative day 1. Suture lines should be kept moist with antibiotic ointment. Sutures and staples are removed sequentially during the first 10 days. Pa-tients experiencing an uneventful recovery can anticipate gradual return to normal activities over a 2- to 4-week period. They should avoid excessive sun exposure and nonsurgical skin treatments (including facials) for the first few months. Exposed and troublesome neck telangi-ectasias (erythroplasia of Queyrat) or bruising can be treated by a V-beam laser at 3 months postoperatively.

It is not unusual for patients to experience firm subcutaneous areas or immature scars during the first year after surgery. These scars should

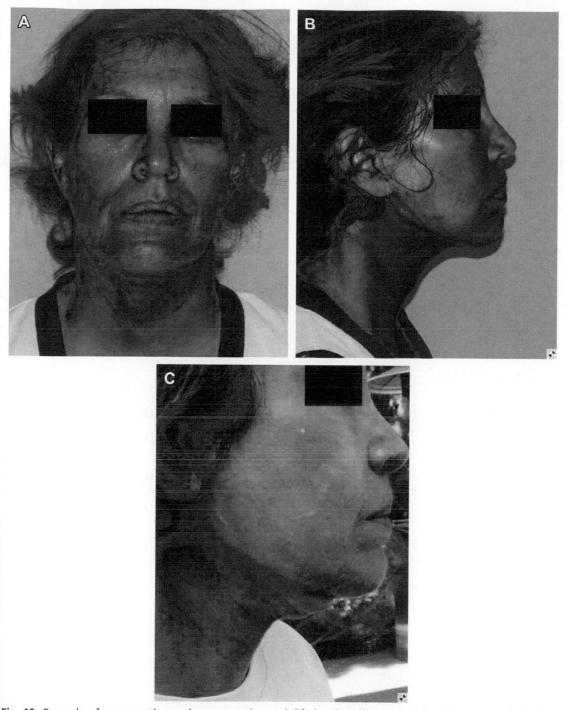

Fig. 10. Example of preoperative and postoperative neck lift (*A, B*). Following a delayed seroma and development of firm contour irregularity (*C*).

be gently massaged by patients or can be treated with ultrasound therapy or injected with triamcinolone 10. Care should be taken to avoid overtreating these localized defects because they tend to resolve spontaneously.

SUMMARY

Isolated surgery of the neck without a facelift is increasingly in demand and a satisfying option for patients concerned with the aging appearance of the neck. It seems to be requested frequently in men and in patients who are satisfied with nonsurgical rejuvenation of the midface or who want to avoid preauricular scars of a facelift operation. Currently, neck surgery probably represents what upper facelift surgery meant to the earlier generation before nonsurgical alternatives were available to treat the midface.

As history has so often shown in surgery, much happens but very little may change. Neck lift surgery is an isolated component of what is performed on the neck during traditional facelift surgery, with modifications in the skin incisions and vector of pull.

REFERENCES

1. Nora Ephron, "I Feel Bad About My Neck" Alfred A. Knopf, New York 2006.
2. Ellenbogen R, Karlin JV. Visual criteria for success in restoring the youthful neck. Plast Reconstr Surg 1980;66(6):826–37.
3. Greer SE, Matarasso A, Wallach S, et al. Importance of the nasal-to-cervical relationship to the profile in rhinoplasty surgery. Plast Reconstr Surg 2001; 108(2):522–31.
4. Matarasso A. Managing the Buccal Fat Pad. Aesthet Surg J 2006;26(3):330–6.
5. Souza Pinto EB. Importance of cervicomental complex treatment in rhytidoplasty. Aesthetic Plast Surg 1981;5(1):69–75.
6. Ellenbogen R. Pseudo-paralysis of the mandibular branch of the facial nerve after platysmal face-lift operation. Plast Reconstr Surg 1979; 63(3):364–8.
7. Guerrerosantos J. Aesthetic necklift. Clin Plast Surg 1983.
8. Connel BF. Neck contour deformities. Clin Plast Surg 1987;14(4):68.

Multidimensional Evaluation and Surgical Approaches to Neck Rejuvenation

Oscar M. Ramirez, MD[a,b],*

KEYWORDS

- Cervicoplasty • Neck aesthetics • Aging neck • Deep cervicoplasty • Neck rejuvenation
- Mandibular implants

KEY POINTS

- Aging of the neck is dependent of: skin elasticity, amount of superficial and deep neck fat accumulation, quality and volume of mandibular support, degenerative changes of the cervical spine and body mass index.
- Evaluation of the neck should take into account the superficial and deep structures as it relates the factors above mentioned.
- The surgical plan to be outlined will depend of the aesthetic and anatomical findings.
- Cervicoplasty should not be limited to the treatment of the skin, subcutaneous fat and platysma muscle only. It should consider the changes in the deep structures of the neck: deep cervical fat, digastrics and salivary gland.
- Assessment of volume and quality of support of the entire mandible should be a routine part of your preoperative evaluation.
- Appropriate surgical maneuvers should be planned based on a comprehensive, multidimensional evaluation.

Editor Commentary: Oscar and I began our friendship in the mid 90's when he was pioneering the endoscopic approach to upper, middle, and lower third facial rejuvenation. His interest in evaluating the anatomical findings in the aging neck and correlating the anatomy to the surgical technique is a common thread throughout his chapter. His advice is logical and intended to safely guide the reader to the best approach to reverse the signs of the aging neck adding ancillary techniques such as suture suspension to improve the outcome.

OVERVIEW

Neck aging is still a challenging problem despite that many procedures and techniques have been described over the years.[1–8] A result that looks good in the early postoperative period can be followed a few weeks or months later with frustrating subcutaneous indurations, skin flaccidity, contour irregularities due to preexisting salivary gland ptosis, digastric "malposition" hypertrophy or subplatysma fat that has not been addressed during the initial surgery. Despite the emphasis of many surgeons on the platysma banding, recurrence of this problem is limited to patients with thin necks.

[a] Private Practice, "Ramirez Plastic Surgery" at Elite Center for Cosmetic Surgery, 2665 Executive Park Drive, Suite 1, Weston, FL 33331, USA; [b] Private Practice, Clinica Corporacion de Cirujanos Plasticos, General Vidal 241, Miraflores, Lima, Peru
* "Ramirez Plastic Surgery" at Elite Center for Cosmetic Surgery, 2665 Executive Park Drive, Suite 1, Weston, FL 33331.
E-mail address: DrRamirez@ramirezmd.com

Clin Plastic Surg 41 (2014) 99–107
http://dx.doi.org/10.1016/j.cps.2013.09.011
0094-1298/14/$ – see front matter © 2014 Elsevier Inc. All rights reserved.

Not all necks are alike. Aesthetic problems of the cervical area are influenced by the following:

- Age
- Inherent skin elasticity
- Subcutaneous and subplatysma fat accumulation
- Volume and quality of the skeletal support of the mandible from the chin to the gonial angle
- Natural height of the cervical spine
- Presence of arthritic changes on the cervical spine that modifies its height and curvature
- Body mass index (BMI)

Aging of the neck is greatly influenced by the acquired or inherent anatomic, aesthetic, and metabolic milieu. An aging neck in the preexisting presence of low BMI with a long slender neck with a normal curvature and excellent mandibular support is going to be completely different from the aging neck in a patient with high BMI, short neck, and poor skeletal support. Between these 2 extremes are a wide variety of conditions that need to be individualized to treat the patient adequately.

In the first situation (low BMI, long slender neck, normal curvature, mandibular support), simpler techniques, such as a cervicofacial lift from the lateral approach, will work well. In the second situation (high BMI, short neck, poor skeletal support), this simple procedure as is proposed by many surgeons will give at best a mediocre result and, at worst, it will make more apparent the underlying anatomic issues with associated aesthetic deformities.

This simple analysis will explain why you cannot compare techniques when you apply them to different anatomic and clinical situations. Any 2 techniques have to be compared when you apply them to similar clinical situations.

Obesity

Obesity is an ever-increasing problem in the United States and in most of the industrialized world with 60 million obese adults in the United States. Likewise, there is increasing rate of obesity in children and teenagers. Since 1980, overweight rates have doubled among children and tripled among adolescents (Centers for Disease Control and Prevention, Behavioral Risk Factor Surveillance System, 2006). That is the population that plastic surgeons will be seeing as patients when they approach middle and old age, not to mention the current middle-age and aging population. Obesity affects not only the trunk but also to a significant degree the face and neck. Those patients develop accumulation

of subcutaneous fat not only on the anterior neck but also on the posterior neck. They also develop fat accumulation deep to the platysma muscle more than average-weight people. Overweight and obese patients also present more jowling. Obesity is a condition essential to consider during preoperative planning.

Bulging Digastric Muscle

Bulging of the anterior belly of digastric muscle is another problem not routinely approached during cervicoplasty. This bulging can be due to hypertrophy or malposition of the muscle. I do not know why hypertrophy occurs. Malposition of the anterior belly of the digastric is related to the low-lying position of the hyoid bone. This is seen in patients with obtuse- firm necks and in patients with microgenia.

Salivary Gland Ptosis

Salivary gland ptosis is another complex problem that affects many patients and makes it difficult to obtain a nice contour on the neck during cervicoplasty. Salivary gland ptosis can happen in patients with thin or heavy necks. Preoperatively it is easier to spot this problem in thin necks. Patients with heavy necks can camouflage minor or large degrees of salivary gland ptosis. This can be a trap for the inexperienced surgeon because, if you overlook diagnosing this condition, postoperatively you will have an unsatisfied patient who will claim that you missed removal of "a lump" of fat tissue, which obviously it is not. Postoperative explanations to an angry patient do not go well and correction of this problem is more complicated at this stage.

Cervical Spine Degeneration

A problem not recognized in the etiology of aesthetic problems of the neck during aging is the gradual shortening of the cervical spine due to arthritic changes and the natural shrinkage or herniations of the intervertebral discs. Those changes are common to the entire length of the spinal column and the cervical spine is not spared of these degenerative processes. This will shorten the entire cervical cylinder, which, in turn, will push the deep neck and floor of the mouth structures to the areas of least resistance, which are the submandibular and submental triangles. As a consequence, the salivary glands, digastric/mylohyoid muscles and the subplatysma fat will "herniate" anteriorly and inferiorly. The more superficial neck envelope, skin, and platysma muscle will also become more redundant in the vertical and horizontal dimensions.

Mandible Skeletal Support

The size of the skeletal support of the mandible also influences how one ages on the lower face and neck. Poor support at the chin, mandibular body, and angle will allow drift of lower face structures into the neck, blunting the submandibular trough and making more obtuse the cervicomental angle. They will also make more apparent the bulging of the submental/submandibular structures.

PREOPERATIVE PLANNING

A careful and comprehensive analysis is important for a good surgical planning. The patient should be made aware of all the issues outlined in the overview: amount of superficial and deep cervical fat, quality of the skeletal support around the chin and mandible, how thick or thin is the entire cervical cylinder, what structures are bulging, if there is salivary gland ptosis or not, how much of skin redundancy exists, the presence or absence of platysma bands, and so forth. Based on these findings, a surgical proposal will be made.

You will need to outline the need to augment the skeletal support, and you will discuss how to treat the deep neck structures and how you will approach the neck. Will you use the lateral approach only or will you also need to use the anterior approach? How will you treat the platysma and skin? These are important considerations because the best cervicoplasty will not give a good result in the absence of good skeletal support. If the patient has heavy, deep structures, a standard cervicoplasty will still have the outcome of a heavy neck postoperatively. Because the management of the salivary gland ptosis is the most complicated and time-consuming proposition, patients need to understand very well the pros and cons of that approach. Many times patients make surgical decisions based on economical factors. He or she has to understand that postoperatively there will be some residuals and sometimes more apparent issues, such as bulging of the salivary gland that he or she did not notice preoperatively (**Figs. 1** and **2**).

When you add more complicated procedures to the standard cervicofacial lift, these will increase the operative time and cost. This is particularly true if you add chin and gonial angle augmentation and a deep cervicoplasty. On many occasions, the components of the planned surgeries may need to be staged to get the best results and avoid prolonged anesthesia time.

Standard preoperative cardiovascular risk evaluation, avoidance of blood thinners, control of hypertension, and so forth is directed in all patients.

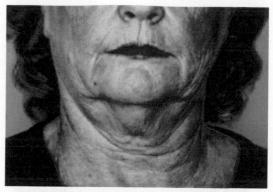

Fig. 1. This patient scheduled for a biplanar facial rejuvenation presents deep neck fullness associated to a salivary gland ptosis and enlargement. She elected not to have salivary gland surgery.

Arrangements for postoperative care under a health care provider, usually a certified nurse with experience in plastic surgery postoperative care is made, particularly if a deep cervicoplasty is done, because of the potential of postoperative bleeding.

Recovery time and time to return to work depends on the extent of the surgery. This can vary from 1 to 4 weeks.

SURGICAL TECHNIQUE
Lateral and Anterior Approach

Most of my patients are approached through lateral and anterior incisions. This is irrespective of age and amount of work you need to do. The reason is that most patients need some work on the anterior neck: platysma, submental fat, and so forth. I have better control of those structures from the submental incision. The submental incision is usually made 1.0 to 1.5 cm posterior to the submental crease. This incision also allows

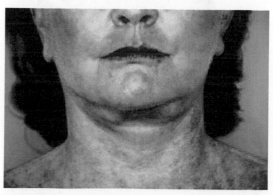

Fig. 2. Postoperatively, despite the improvement obtained at every other level, she presents accentuation of the salivary gland fullness.

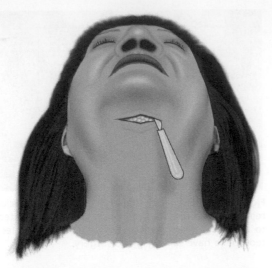

Fig. 3. The submental incision for the anterior approach is made 1.0 to 1.5 cm posterior to the submental crease.

me to perform a subcutaneous/subdermal dissection from this incision to the anterior lower chin and separate the attachments of the skin to the submental crease and prejowl ligaments. This dissection tends to be bloody and I can control this subdermal bleeding better from this approach. This dissection allows better redraping of the perimental skin. This submental incision also allows you to advance the platysma medially and move the skin in the opposite direction. Logistically,

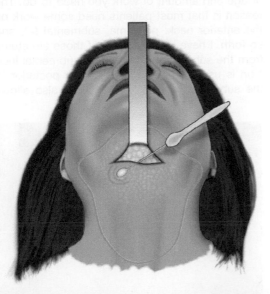

Fig. 4. A wide subcutaneous undermining is done via the submental approach. At least 0.5-cm subcutaneous fat thickness should be preserved under the dermis.

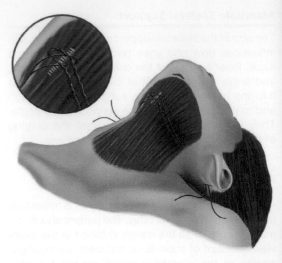

Fig. 5. Showing the interlocked Giampapa cervical suture suspension (GSS).

you cannot do that if you use the lateral approach exclusively.

Lateral Approach

Obviously, there will be exceptions in which there is not a need to do these maneuvers and you can handle everything from the lateral approach. The lateral approach exclusively is indicated in patients with the following:

- Smooth submental crease area
- Absence of submental bulge
- Absence of platysma bands

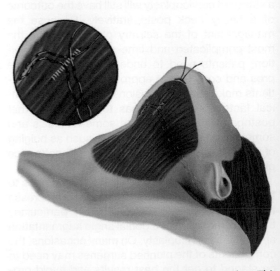

Fig. 6. The Ramirez Pursestring suture suspension. This is a variation of the GSS. The double row of sutures are woven into the platysma. This maneuver recruits muscle over the salivary gland for enhanced support while it takes care of the platysma redundancy.

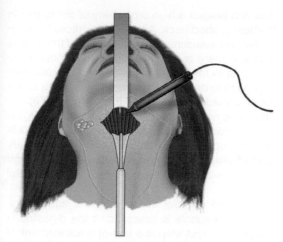

Fig. 7. When approaching the deep neck compartment the platysma is opened vertically from pogonium to cricoid cartilage level.

- Absence of visible prejowl dimples

On the other hand, I use the submental incision exclusively in young or middle-age patients who do not have too much excess of skin and most of the problems are in the submental area (**Figs. 3** and **4**). The rest of the neck can be remodeled with liposuction and a suture suspension

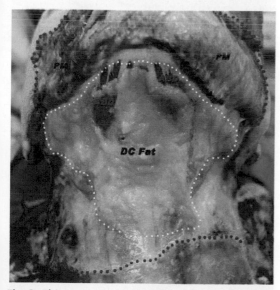

Fig. 8. This anatomical preparation shows the deep cervical fat compartment. This typically has a trapezoidal shape and extends beyond the level of the salivary glands laterally. Red dots indicate level of platysma muscle division. Blue mark on the specimen: bony attachment of playsma muscle. White dotted line indicate the boundaries of the deep cervical fat. ABD, anterior belly of digastric; DC Fat, Deep Cervical fat; PM, platysma muscle lifted above and over the mandible.

applied through a retroauricular/mastoid mini-incision, as described by Giampapa and DiBernardo (**Fig. 5**).[9] If there is excess skin, this can be redraped posteriorly with through-and-through skin undermining using mini-incisions in the retroauricular/occipital scalp and applying the Ramirez modification of the Giampapa suture suspension (**Fig. 6**). This requires an endoscope for accurate dissection and control of bleeding.[10] Mentopexy and/or chin implants will also dictate the need for an anterior incision.

Neck Fat and Neck Bulge

Neck defatting is done by direct trimming with scissors via the submental approach. I do liposuction only when an entirely closed approach is used or as a way to debulk a heavy subcutaneous fat accumulation and I do the fine contouring with the scissors. The decision to resect interdigastric/subplatysma fat is usually made intraoperatively.

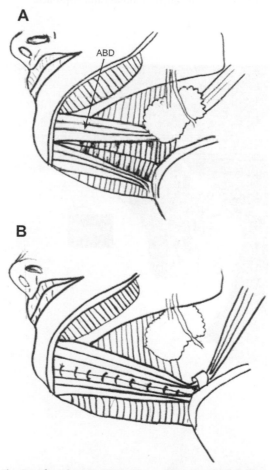

Fig. 9. After the interdigastric and the rest of the deep cervical fat resection the anterior belly of digastrics (ABD) can be sutured as a corset in the midline. A: before the digastric corset. B: after the digastric corset.

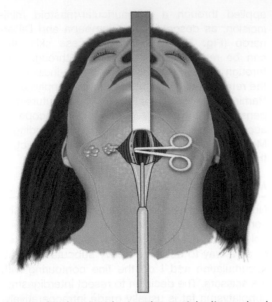

Fig. 10. This drawing depicts the partial salivary gland resection via the central subplatysma approach.

You can predict a high probability of doing this in the heavy, short neck. After the superficial fat is resected, an assessment of the contour of the neck is made. If there is bulging, a decision to open the platysma in the midline is made and a graduated approach to deal with the deep subplatysma structures is made starting with the deep fat (**Fig. 7**). This fat is not confined to the interdigastric region only. It has a trapezoidal shape and it extends laterally up to the area underlying the salivary glands (**Fig. 8**).[11] If you resect only the central part you will develop a hollowed out submental area.

Next, the contour of the digastric against the mylohyoid muscle is assessed. If the digastric is bulging, the first step is a trial of advancement of this muscle toward the midline. If that fills the gap and the contour is improved, then a corset of the anterior belly of the digastrics (ABD) with inverted sutures using 3-0 nylon is made (**Fig. 9**). If

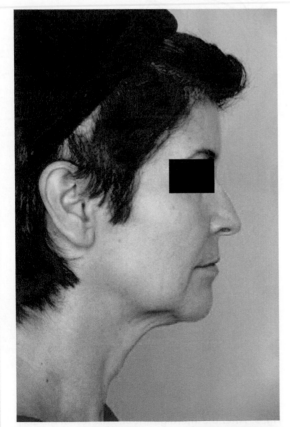

Fig. 11. Preoperative view of this 55-year-old female. She has obtuse cervicomental angle with skin and platysma muscle redundancy and bands.

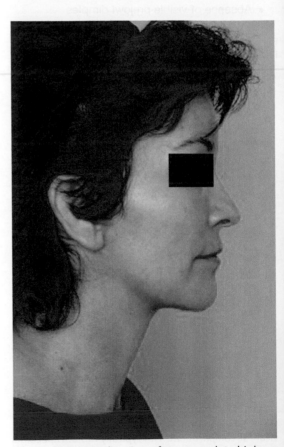

Fig. 12. Postoperative view after a complete biplanar endoscopic assisted mask (BEAM) facial rejuvenation. Observe the smooth, clean and well defined neck and cervicomental angle. The patient had a bidirectional approach to the neck rejuvenation. The platysma corset was complemented with the Ramirez Woven Suture Suspension.

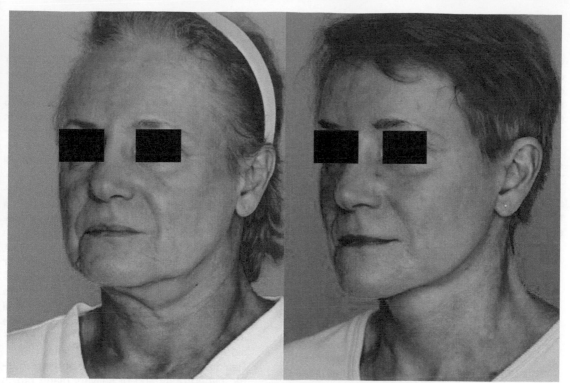

Fig. 13. Before and after of a patient with a TEAM (triplanar endoscopic-assisted mask) facial rejuvenation. This included the subplatysma deep cervicoplasty with partial salivary excision on the left.

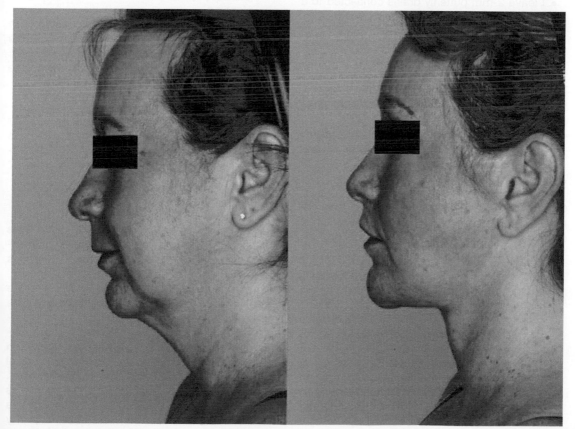

Fig. 14. Before and after of a patient with the TEAM facial rejuvenation. The obtuse neck treatment required subplatysma deep neck cervicoplasty with DC fat excision and a geniomandibular Ramirez (RZ) medpor chin implant.

that does not improve it, then a tangential shaving of the superficial portion of the ABD is done. If preoperatively enlarged ptotic salivary glands are detected or during surgery the glands are bulging, the superficial lobe of the gland is removed on each side (**Fig. 10**).

Cervicoplasty

To perform deep cervicoplasty, long slender instruments are needed. I usually use 2 lighted retractors and commonly do bleeding control with small hemoclips.

- The platysma muscle is closed after they are advanced to the midline.
- If the platysma is thin, I do not resect the redundancy. I will overlap or fold the edges as I apply the interrupted sutures from the mentum to the hyoid.
- In cases of platysma banding, I usually do 2 Z-plasties of the anterior 4 cm of the muscle. I handle the redundant muscle with the Ramirez pursestring woven suture suspension and/or I resect the muscle in the lowest part of the dissected area.
- I leave 2-mm butterfly drains connected to a vacutainer tubes, one on each side of the sub-platysma plane and one on each side of the superficial plane. I do not use fibrin glue. I advance the drains on the second or third day and I usually remove them on the fifth or sixth day, a bit longer than the standard. This allows me to suction all the potential seroma that may form.
- Following these steps, you can obtain reliable and consistent excellent results (**Figs. 11–14**).

SEQUELA AND COMPLICATIONS

Complications and sequelae following cervicoplasty can range from a simple nuisance to a devastating problem.

- Injury to one or more branches of the marginal mandibular nerve (MMN) can be devastating to the patient. Luckily this is rarely permanent. Recovery of the nerve can be hastened with electrical myoneural stimulation. Avoidance of aggressive liposuction or avoidance of monopolar cautery around the trajectory of the MMN will minimize this risk.
- Acute hematoma in a closed compartment can be a life-threatening complication. Any hypertension should be controlled and patients should be watched carefully, particularly in the first 24 hours. During surgery, hemostasis should be precise with bipolar

or coaxial suction coagulator. A large or medium-size vessel should be ligated with sutures or hemoclips.
- Subdermal/subcutaneous indurations due to seromas or hematomas can be resolved with serial injections of diluted triamcinolone. Prevention of seromas includes prevention of hematomas and the use of close-system small drains for several days.
- Contour irregularities from residual fat accumulations can be corrected with liposuction by using small cannulas. This can be prevented with meticulous contouring with the sharp scissors.
- Skin necrosis resulting from smoking or excessive tension requires a secondary correction after the area has been allowed to heal and the skin left to soften for several months. Prevention includes perioperative avoidance of smoking and control of skin tension during closure.
- Residual bulging due to anterior belly of digastric hypertrophy and or salivary gland ptosis requires a secondary deep cervicoplasty. Avoidance of these problems requires a good preoperative assessment and surgical planning.
- Small areas of residual platysma banding can be improved with botox injections. Large areas will require secondary platysmaplasty. To avoid residual platysma banding, the appropriate technique should be used: muscle z-plasty, muscle back cut, and so forth.

In general, the timing of any revision is better done after you wait the longest. The minimum is 6 months, ideally 12 months. However, psychological issues may determine earlier revision.

SUMMARY

Correction of aesthetic and anatomic deformities of the neck due to aging is a complex proposition, and the planning and approach depends on the findings during your initial examination. Surgical techniques need to be adapted to the problems you encounter.[12] More than any area of the body, an in-depth knowledge of the anatomy is mandatory. The surgery can be very simple or highly technical. Surgeons should have in their armamentarium all the available surgical techniques to provide the best aesthetic result. The deep cervicoplasty is not the same as the superficial cervicoplasty; it is completely a different surgical dimension. Deep cervicoplasty is not for the occasional facial rejuvenative surgeon. You require experience in diagnosing neck problems, executing the proper surgical maneuvers, and effectively tackling acute and late complications.

REFERENCES

1. Owsley JQ Jr. SMAS-platysma facelift. A bidirectional cervicofacial rhytidectomy. Clin Plast Surg 1983;10(3):429–40.
2. Labbe D, Franco RG, Nicolas J. Platysma suspension and platysmaplasty during neck lift: anatomical study an analysis of 30 cases. Plast Reconstr Surg 2006;117(6):2001–7.
3. Millard DR Jr, Garst WP, Beck RL, et al. Submental and submandibular lipectomy in conjunction with face lift, in the male or female. Plast Reconstr Surg 1972;49(4):385–91.
4. Fuente del Campo A. Midline platysma muscular overlap for neck restoration. Plast Reconstr Surg 1998;102(5):1710–4.
5. Ramirez OM. Cervicoplasty: non-excisional anterior approach. Plast Reconstr Surg 1997;99:1576–85.
6. Ramirez OM, Robertson KM. Comprehensive approach to rejuvenation of the neck. Facial Plast Surg 2001;17(2):129–40.
7. Giampapa VC, Bitzos I, Ramirez OM, et al. Suture suspension platysmaplasty for neck rejuvenation revisited: technical fine points for improving outcomes. Aesthetic Plast Surg 2005; 29(5):341–50.
8. Giampapa VC, Bitzos I, Ramirez OM, et al. Long-term results of suture suspension platysmaplasty for neck rejuvenation: a 13-year follow-up evaluation. Aesthetic Plast Surg 2005;29(5):332–40.
9. Giampapa VC, DiBernardo BE. Neck recontouring with suture suspension and liposuction: an alternative for the early rhytidectomy candidate. Aesthetic Plast Surg 1995;19(3):217–23.
10. Ramirez OM. Cervicoplasty without skin excision. In: Shiffman MA, Mirrafati SJ, Lam SM, et al, editors. Simplified facial rejuvenation. Berlin: Springer Verlag; 2008. p. 613–20 Chapter 80.
11. Ramirez OM. Advanced considerations determining procedure selection in cervicoplasty. Part one: anatomy and aesthetics. Clin Plast Surg 2008;35(4):679–90.
12. Ramirez OM. Advanced considerations determining procedure selection in cervicoplasty. Part two: surgery. Clin Plast Surg 2008;35(4):691–709.

Neck Rejuvenation With Suture Suspension Platysmaplasty Technique
A Minimally Invasive Neck Lift Technique That Addresses All Patients' Anatomic Needs

Vincent C. Giampapa, MD, FACS[a],*, John M. Mesa, MD[b,c]

KEYWORDS

- Neck lift • Neck rejuvenation • Platysmaplasty • Suture suspension • Minimally invasive neck lift

KEY POINTS

- The suture suspension platysmaplasty neck lift creates a permanent artificial "ligament" under the mandible, correcting the deformities of the aging neck.
- The suture suspension platysmaplasty technique suspends the midline platysma muscle and displaces the lateral platysma muscle under the border of the mandible in a natural way.
- Fixation of the suture on the mastoid fascia with the appropriate tension is an essential step in this procedure.
- Extremely careful analysis of the 6 points of neck rejuvenation and customization of the suture suspension platysmaplasty technique according to these points allows the aesthetic surgeon to fully rejuvenate the neck with a long-lasting result.
- This technique is simple, safe, and reproducible, with excellent patient satisfaction outcomes.

Editor Commentary: Vince Giampapa first published his suture suspension technique in 1995. His technique has evolved with the important addition of a submandibular angle loop suture to his suspension technique that improves the aesthetic appearance of the neck while decreasing the tension on the suspension suture. His algorithm is also important in deciding which candidates can be managed by suture suspension alone. Many surgeons add his technique or a variation of it to their neck-lifting procedure to improve the cervicomental angle. Probably many of us wish we had added this procedure when we feel that our postoperative neck contour could have been better.

INTRODUCTION

Neck rejuvenation has been one of the most important components in the treatment for the aging face because the neck is frequently the first feature to show the signs of aging.[1] The aging neck is characterized by the development of an obtuse cervicomental angle, elimination of the smooth jawline border, appearance of vertical neck bands, and accumulation of submental fat and excess skin. The ideal neck surgical rejuvenation technique should correct all of these findings with minimal morbidity and short downtime.

Multiple techniques have been described to perform neck lifts as an isolated procedure or in conjunction with a rhytidectomy.[2-4] In 1973, Guerrero-Santos and colleagues[2] described the

[a] Division of Plastic and Reconstructive Surgery, Rutgers University, Newark, New Jersey, USA; [b] Division of Plastic Surgery, University of Alabama at Birmingham, Birmingham, Alabama, USA; [c] Private Practice, Plastic Surgery Center Internationale, Montclair, New Jersey, USA
* Corresponding author.
E-mail address: giampapamd@aol.com

Clin Plastic Surg 41 (2014) 109–124
http://dx.doi.org/10.1016/j.cps.2013.09.005
0094-1298/14/$ – see front matter © 2014 Elsevier Inc. All rights reserved.

muscular lift. Feldman[3] described the corset platysmaplasty in 1989. In 1990, Giampapa and Di Bernardo[5] developed the concept of the suture-suspension neck lift; initially performed in patients with open facelift, and later performed as a closed neck lift approach. Long-term evaluation of the suture suspension technique has shown that this technique gives the patient a long-lasting rejuvenation of the neck, especially in the cervicomental angle.[6]

Suture suspension platysmaplasty is a powerful, versatile, and minimally invasive technique for neck rejuvenation that addresses the aging neck with minimal morbidity and short postsurgical "downtime."[7]

INDICATIONS FOR PLATYSMAPLASTY

Neck rejuvenation with suture suspension platysmaplasty is indicated for virtually any patient with signs of neck aging.[7,8] Obtaining benefits from this powerful surgical technique are both old and young patients with the following:

- Obtuse cervicomental angle
- Absence of smooth jawline border
- Presence of vertical neck bands (platysma bands)
- Accumulation of submental fat and excess of neck skin

Suture suspension platysmaplasty neck lift could be performed alone or in conjunction with facelift (**Fig. 1**). This is especially important in patients who, for medical or economic reasons, do not wish to undergo a facelift at the same time of a neck lift. Additionally, performing neck rejuvenation without the traditional preauricular facelift incision is appealing to the male patient population.

An appropriate candidate for this procedure should meet several of the following criteria:

1. Poorly defined cervicomental angle
2. Poorly defined submandibular border
3. Absence of laxity in the midface structures (because no tightening of the underlying superficial musculoaponeurotic system fibers and facial muscles in the midface is accomplished through this procedure)
4. Mild to moderate amount of jowling and neck fat (those with large amounts of neck and jowl

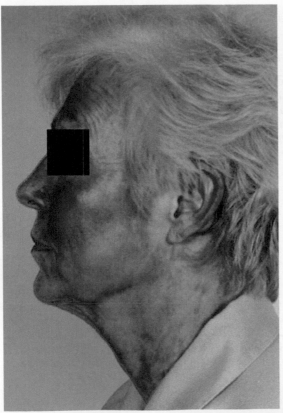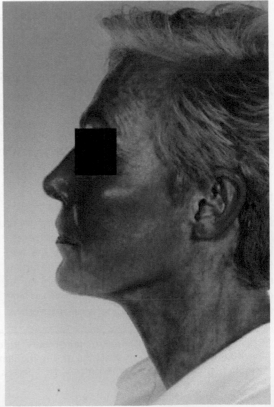

Fig. 1. Suture suspension platysmaplasty neck lift performed alone or in conjunction with facelift.

fat will find some soft tissue irregularities if this procedure is used alone in lieu of a facelift)

5. Unwillingness or inability to undergo a full facelift

Although the suture suspension surgical technique seems to fit a wide range of patients with an aging neck, there is a specific group of patients that will not fully benefit from it: those patients with severe midface laxity and severe jowls will not achieve the desired and expected results with this technique alone (**Tables 1** and **2**). This specific subgroup of patients *requires concomitant midface lifting* (preauricular incision) to address the excess of skin and adipose tissue at the lower face/neck junction (severe jowls) that would mask the results of suture suspension neck lift.[9]

SYSTEMATIC NECK EVALUATION FOR SUTURE SUSPENSION PLATYSMAPLASTY NECK LIFT

The outcomes of any neck rejuvenation surgical technique rely importantly in the careful preoperative assessment of the neck deformities associated with aging. We have carefully described 6 basic anatomic points of the neck rejuvenation.[8] These 6 anatomic points must be carefully and systematically analyzed to personalize the suture suspension platysmaplasty to perfectly fit the patient's needs and therefore achieve an outstanding and desired aesthetic outcome.

Our 6 basic anatomic points for the neck rejuvenation are the following:

1. Cervicomental angle
2. Mandibular border definition
3. Mandibular angle definition
4. Labiomandibular fold prominence ("jowls")
5. Mental (chin) prominence
6. Anterior neck width

DESCRIPTION OF THE 6 KEY ANATOMIC POINTS OF NECK REJUVENATION
Point 1: Cervicomental Angle

The cervicomental angle is one of the fundamental determinants of the youthful neck (**Fig. 2**). The cervicomental angle is usually between 105° and 120°. Change of this angle to a more obtuse one is an early and strong sign of neck aging. Cervicomental angle depth is limited by the patient's anatomy. To evaluate the neck with the patient in an interactive manner, we suggest taking a long cotton swab, or something long and thin, and pressing against the neck line to show how deep the cervicomental angle is (ie, the distance between the anterior-most tip of the mentum and the thyroid cartilage). This maneuver done in front of the mirror will show the patient the amount of realistic improvement expected from a neck lift. In people with a narrow neck, even the best neck lift may not yield a dramatic improvement if the patient's expectations are unrealistic.

Point 2: Mandibular Border Definition

One of the goals of a neck lift is to re-create the mandibular contour by repositioning the platysma and tucking it underneath the border of the mandible (**Fig. 3**). With a wider and more prominent jaw, we obtain better results. One of the initial questions in a consultation is, "Does the patient have a nice, full, wide jaw, or is it narrow?" If the patient has a narrow jaw, the results are not going to be as dramatic as in an individual with a wide jaw. Patients of Romanian or Slavic descent who have wide jaws do very well with a neck lift.

Table 1
Classification of neck types according to anatomic finding versus appropriate neck rejuvenation surgical technique

| Anatomic Finding | Neck Type Classification | | | |
	I	II	III	IV
Midface	No laxity	Mild	Moderate	Severe
Jowls	None	Mild	Moderate	Severe (prominent)
Submental fat accumulation	Mild	Moderate	Moderate	Severe
Platysma laxity	Mild	Moderate	Moderate	Moderate to severe
Treatment	Suture suspension platysmaplasty or SAL alone	Suture suspension platysmaplasty	Suture suspension platysmaplasty	Facelift + suture suspension platysmaplasty

Abbreviation: SAL, suction assisted lipectomy.

Table 2
The 6 key anatomic points of neck rejuvenation and their surgical correction

Anatomic Point	Description	Correction of the Deficiency
1	Cervicomental angle	• Adjusting the tension of the interlocking suspension suture • Defatting supraplatysmal and subplatysmal space • Suturing the digastric muscles together • Transecting platysma borders
2	Mandibular border definition	• SAL above and below the border of the mandibular border (leaving a strip of subcutaneous fat along the bony border) • Fat grafting to the mandibular border • Long-term fillers (eg, HA-based fillers)
3	Mandibular angle definition	• Loop suture (of the suture suspension platysmaplasty) at the sternocleidomastoid muscle under the angle of the mandible • Fat grafting into masseter • Long-term soft tissue fillers at the angle of mandible (eg, HA filler) • Alloplastic mandibular angle augmentation
4	Labiomandibular fold prominence ("jowls")	• SAL of jowls from submental and postauricular approaches • Camouflage fat grafting • Depressor labii muscle release • Barbed sutures ("threat lift suture")
5	Mental prominence (chin)	• Alloplastic chin augmentation • Fat grafting to the chin • Long-term fillers
6	Anterior neck width	• Resection and medial advancement of platysma muscle along full length of neck • Imbrications of platysma muscle in the midline • SAL of prominent subcutaneous fat

Abbreviation: SAL, suction assisted lipectomy.

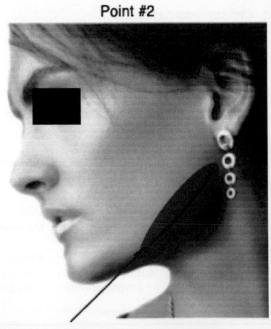

Point #1

Point #2

Fig. 2. Point 1: cervicomental angle.

Fig. 3. Point 2: mandibular border definition.

Northern Europeans with narrow faces or Latin Americans with smaller facial features may not have as good a result. Of course these are generalities and exceptions are found.

Point 3: Mandibular Angle Definition

Mandibular angle definition is an important landmark of the neck rejuvenation that is often forgotten by common surgical techniques (**Fig. 4**). A well-defined mandibular angle complements the mandibular border and gives a youthful appearance to the neck. In men, a well-defined and prominent mandibular angle significantly gives a youthful and masculine appearance to the neck and lower face.

Point 4: Labiomandibular Fold Prominence ("Jowls")

Evaluating the midface is very important for a potential neck lift patient (**Fig. 5**). Minimal laxity to midface structures is important in achieving a good neck lift. At the initial consultation, it should be made clear to the patient that a neck lift is not the procedure of choice to improve the jowls or the nasolabial folds. It is recommended to pinch the patients' jowls to remind them, physically, that this area will not be improved significantly with a neck lift. This point cannot be overemphasized because patients may feel that they will get all the benefits of a facelift with a neck lift, but with "less surgery." That is not true, especially if the patient has significant jowls. A neck lift is

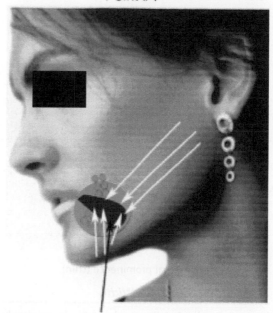

Point #4

Fig. 5. Point 4: labiomandibular fold prominence ("jowls").

meant to make a new cervicomental angle and new definition, but is it not a substitute for a facelift, especially when addressing the jowls in a person with significant midface laxity (see **Table 1**). There is the occasional patient who comes back after surgery and says, "My neck looks great, but what about this" (pointing to the jowls), and we, as surgeons, remind them of discussing that specific point preoperatively. They acknowledge that fact when they remember the preoperative pinch to that area.

Point 5: Mental Prominence (Chin)

Using a very simple technique, by drawing a vertical line from the glabella down through the upper lip and a second vertical line from the nasal tip to the chin prominence, will help to quickly define whether the chin is normal, hyperplastic, or hypoplastic (**Fig. 6**). A 3-mm to 4-mm augmentation is usually recommended. If the implant is 3 to 4 mm in projection, there is another 2 mm of projection from the soft tissues, which should be enough to balance the chin, except for severe cases of retrusion. That 4 to 5 mm is enough to take up extra skin and give the female jaw a more aesthetically pleasing profile. With men, it is desirable to have a chin augmentation that surpasses the vertical line beyond the lower lip to give a more masculine look.

Point #3

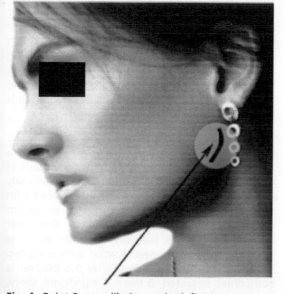

Fig. 4. Point 3: mandibular angle definition.

Point #5

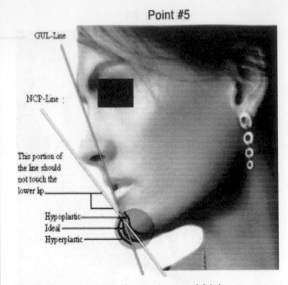

Fig. 6. Point 5: mental prominence (chin).

Point 6: Anterior Neck Width

In many patients, the neck width is markedly increased with aging (**Fig. 7**). This increase is mainly attributable to muscle laxity, collapse of the cervical spine, and an increase in subcutaneous and submental fat deposits.

SUTURE SUSPENSION PLATYSMAPLASTY NECK LIFT SURGICAL TECHNIQUE
Preoperative Management

Patients should get medical and psychiatric clearance when appropriate before proceeding to surgery. It is a good idea to give prospective patients references of people who have had the surgery and consented to be used as references, so the prospective patient may contact them by phone and ask them questions. After the patient is ready for surgery, the immediate preoperative preparation commences. Optimizing a patient for surgery is done differently by surgeons. Some useful steps have been to place patients on vitamin K and Arnica for 5 days preoperatively, requesting that the patients stop taking aspirin and aspirin products for 10 days, and that they abstain from smoking for 2 weeks preoperatively and 2 weeks postoperatively.

Anesthesia

The procedure could be performed under general anesthesia, intravenous sedation, or pure local anesthesia.[10]

Suction-Assisted Lipectomy of the Neck

After the tumescent solution has taken effect, the neck is liposuctioned initially with 2-mm to 3-mm

Point #6

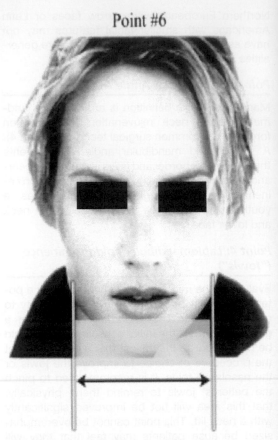

Fig. 7. Point 6: anterior neck width.

spatulated cannulas and finally with a 4-mm liposuction spatulated cannula. The area of the submandibular tunnel is suctioned along its dermal surface with the 4-mm cannula facing the dermis. This maneuver helps encourage skin contraction in this area. Specific areas, such as the anterior border of the sternocleidomastoid, the jowls, and the angle of the mandible, are liposuctioned in the appropriate patient. The inferior border of the liposuction area depends on the amount of fat in the lower aspect of the neck. At times, the whole extent of the neck needs to be suctioned if there is a significant fatty layer.

Management of Platysma Muscle

A midline curvilinear submental incision is made in the horizontal crease, and the skin immediately overlying the platysma muscles is elevated with facelift scissors. A curvilinear incision seems to heal better than a straight incision after scar contraction. Excess subplatysmal fatty tissue is excised under direct visualization with a lighted retractor. The platysma border in the midline is sometimes resected, if there is significant laxity, in a triangular fashion, and the platysma borders are cauterized. Prominent platysma bands are transected for approximately 2 to 3 cm on each side of the platysma border or are imbricated at the midline with suture.

Placement of the Interlocking Suture Suspension ("Artificial Ligament Placement")

At the depth desired to create the new cervicomental angle, usually the hyoid bone, a 3-0 Prolene suture for women or 0 Prolene suture for men is placed in a horizontal mattress fashion from right to left, including both borders of the platysma muscle. Another similar suture is placed from left to right in a vertical mattress style interlocking with the first suture. The ends of both sutures are taken out through the submental incision and the sutures are clamped separately with a Webster needle holder to avoid weakening the suture. The postauricular skin on each side is identified and an ellipse of skin is excised. This maneuver eliminates the redundant skin from the neck in an easily hidden incision and allows better access to the underlying mastoid fascia. The skin between the mastoid area and the submental area is then undermined to connect to the previously made tunnel. A long curved hemostat is placed at the postauricular sulcus and exits through the tunnel at the submental incision. The left suture is grasped by the instrument and taken through the submandibular tunnel. Then, the suture is sutured deep into the mastoid fascia while the patient's face is turned toward the opposite side and maximally extended. The suture is then tied just enough so that the platysma muscle is tucked up underneath the border of the mandible. Similarly, the vertical mattress suture is tied to the right mastoid. The suspension sutures result in a superior and internal vector force that creates the new cervicomental angle and defines the submandibular border (**Fig. 8**). The inherent properties of soft tissue contraction allow the overlying skin to adapt to the new muscle positions.

The Submandibular Angle Loop Suture

An important technical fine point that evolved over the past 15 years is the submandibular angle loop suture.[8] This involves securing the nonabsorbable interlocking suture under the area of the angle of the mandible at the anterior sternocleidomastoid border, before suturing it on the mastoid fascia (**Figs. 9** and **10**). After the loop has been created, the suture is secured at the mastoid process periosteum, and it is critical to keep the tension of the interlocking suture moderate. The suture should be placed on each side of the mastoid fascia while the patient's face is turned toward the opposite side and maximally extended. The angle loop suture creates a more natural and anatomically pleasing result. Additionally, it creates a "hinge mechanism," owing to its geometry, which decreases the suture tension, especially when the patient turns the neck sideways. This eliminates the chance of "overcorrection," and the feeling of tightness that a small percentage of patients experienced before this technical modification was introduced.

Skin Excision

Usually, only a small amount of skin needs to be excised in the form of an elliptical skin strip that extends from the ear lobule area to the midlevel of the postauricular sulcus. It is important to understand that although a fatty neck appears to have too much skin, that this is, in essence, an illusion.

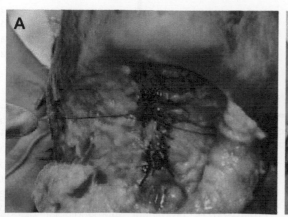
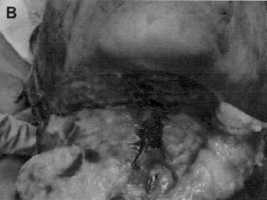

Fig. 8. Cadaver dissection showing the effect of the suture suspension on cervicomental angle. (*A*) Interlocked suture suspension in place at the level of the hyoid without tension. (*B*) Interlocked suture suspension in place at the level of the hyoid with tension.

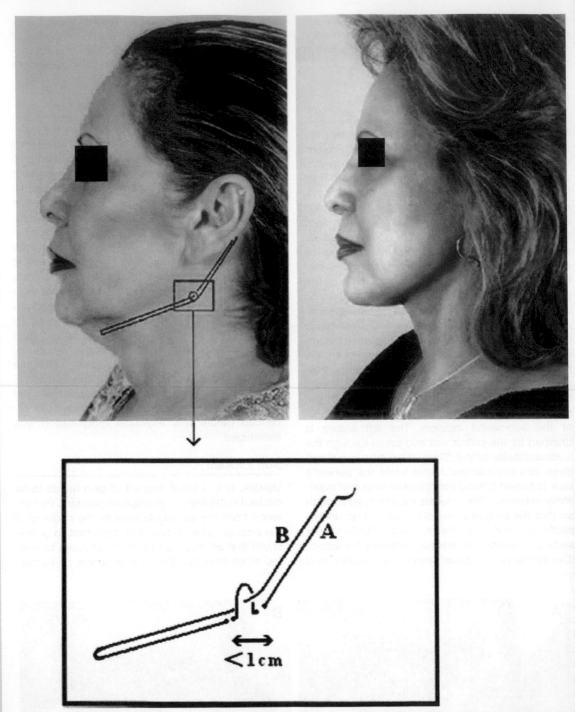

Fig. 9. The "loop angle suture" at the level of the sternocleidomastoid muscle, just below the angle of the mandible to enhance the angle of the mandible. Bottom: diagram of the suture loop. Top left: preoperative. Top right: postoperative.

In reality, a full neck has too little skin rather than too much, owing to the fact that when the cervicomental angle is augmented, and a concavity is subsequently created, more skin is required to fill this.

Management of Submandibular Glands

Prolapsed or prominent submandibular glands can be a problem and need to be addressed initially with the patient, before the surgery. The

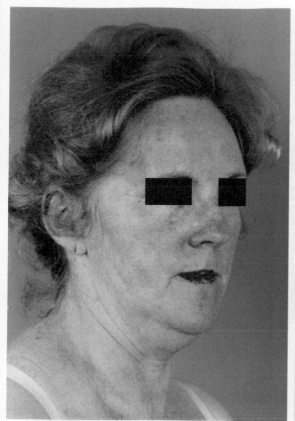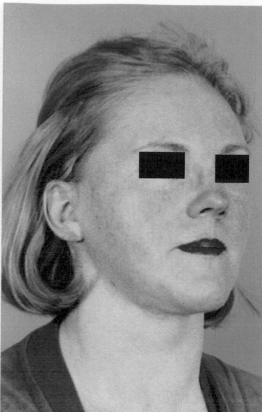

Fig. 10. Surgical correction of Point 1: cervicomental angle.

patient has to be told that even with a good neck lift technique, if he or she has prolapsed or prominent submandibular glands, the result will not be as optimal. Ptotic submandibular glands need to be pointed out to the patient and a discussion about the attempt to improve the contour should be undertaken preoperatively. To demonstrate the location and size of the submandibular gland, a long cotton swab is placed at the cervicomental angle and pressed. The patient feels where the submandibular gland is and can see the outline in a mirror. If the submandibular glands are not shown to the patient preoperatively, when the neck laxity may be masking the glands, then the patient may be dissatisfied with a good result because the "bulge" is more evident after the fat has been liposuctioned and the skin and muscles have been tightened. It is not recommended to resect the submandibular glands, owing to a high complication rate. After the platysmaplication has been performed, the prominent gland prolapses inferiorly. This is called the "hammock effect": If a person sits in a hammock, there is a hanging effect because the weight is great, the hammock is weak, or a combination of both. With the submandibular gland sitting above the platysma, the

analogy holds true. When the suspension suture is placed, the muscle is holding up the gland. A second 3.0 Prolene interlocking suspension suture is placed adjacent to the initial suture, passing inferiorly to the submandibular gland, and tied to the mastoid fascia through the same tunnel where the first suture suspension was placed. The result is the reinforcement of the weak area with a "hammock effect," resulting in the superior elevation of the submandibular gland.

Specific Management of the Key 6 Anatomic Points of Neck Rejuvenation

Surgical correction of point 1: cervicomental angle

Cervicomental angle depth is limited by the patient's anatomy. A number of options exist for enhancing this point. First, placement of the interlocking suspension suture allows for a superior and internal vector that elevates the platysma muscle into its new position, usually immediately above the hyoid. Adjustment of the tension on this suture allows for adjustment of the angle depth from mild to moderate (**Fig. 11**). This factor is discussed in detail preoperatively with the

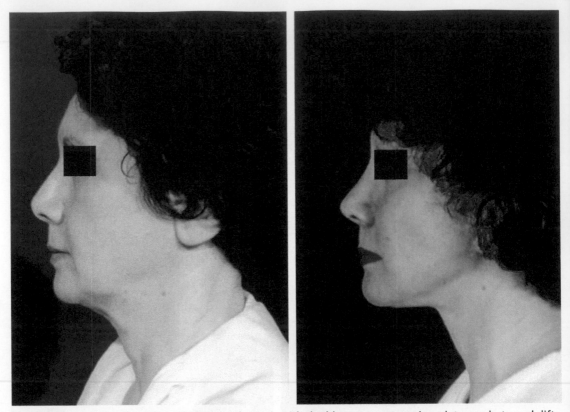

Fig. 11. Management of submandibular glands ptosis with double suture suspension platysmaplasty neck lift.

patient, and a decision is made according to the individual anatomy and the patient's wishes. Additionally, defatting of the supraplatysmal and subplatysmal fat also can enhance this angle or help it remain soft, depending on the effort during the dissection in this area. Special liposuction cannulas (spatula shaped) are used for this purpose with varying degrees of suctioning, again, according the individual anatomy. It is crucial to avoid the "overcorrected neck," which occurs if too much fat is removed from the supraplatysmal or subplatysmal plane, or if too much tension is applied to the suspension sutures. Suturing the digastric muscles together can further enhance the angle and help create a more concave or flat submental triangle. Finally, transection of the platysmal muscle borders medially has been popular, but use of this technique has rarely been found necessary except for patients with extremely thick platysmal bands or severe medial redundancy.

Surgical correction of point 2: mandibular border definition
The key elements of this step in the neck procedure involve suctioning both above and below the border of the mandible and leaving a strip of subcutaneous fat along the bony mandibular

border for highlighting of the border itself (**Fig. 12**). The suctioning along the lower border of the mandible is accomplished by using a spatula cannula to suction both exposed surfaces (platysmal and dermal fat) gently to help enhance the submandibular definition. Additional tools for this anatomic point are fat grafting along the border of the mandible during the primary platysmaplasty, or long-term fillers, such as hyaluronic acid–based fillers. These tools have been used with excellent results, especially for mandibles that are relatively hypoplastic (narrow jaw configuration).

Surgical correction of point 3: mandibular angle definition
Modification of the suspension suture to create a loop immediately before placement of the suture through the mastoid fascia has resulted in extremely well-defined mandibular angles (**Fig. 13**). This is done by taking a small bite of the sternocleidomastoid muscle immediately below the angle of the mandible, then coming out and taking a second bite, thereby creating a loop with the suture. The other end of the suture is placed through the loop, as illustrated in **Fig. 9**. The suspension suture is then placed to the mastoid fascia with the

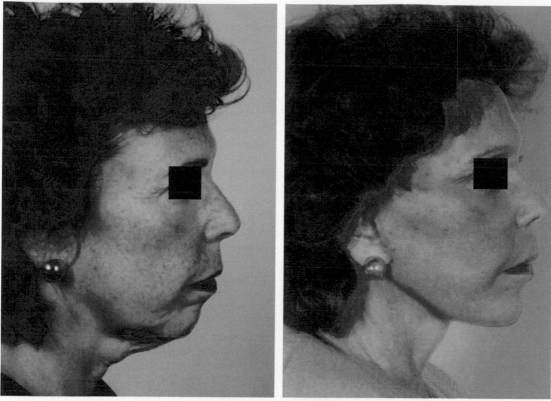

Fig. 12. Surgical correction of Point 2: mandibular border definition.

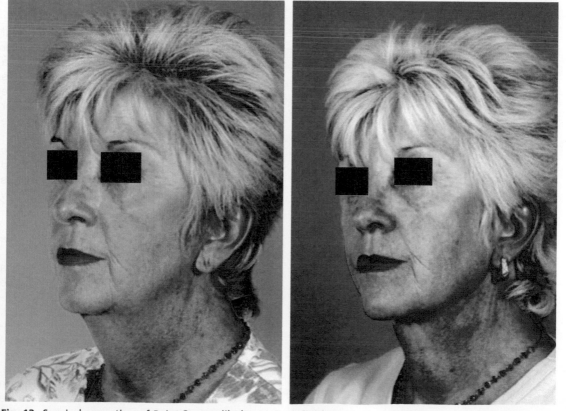

Fig. 13. Surgical correction of Point 3: mandibular angle definition.

appropriate tension (moderate). Additionally, fat grafting into the masseter muscle has resulted in even more defined mandibular angles. The same results were observed when long-term, such as hyaluronic-based fillers, were injected into the inferior mandibular border or the superolateral ramus. Alloplastic augmentation, another alternative, can be performed simultaneously or as another separate procedure.[11]

Surgical correction of point 4: labiomandibular fold prominence ("jowls")

Labiomandibular fold prominence is frequently considered above the neck proper, but it in essence contributes directly to an overall youthful and clean appearance of the neck. Suctioning of this area both from below the submental incision and from the postauricular incision allows for a bilateral vector force resulting in skin contracture in a superolateral direction with consequent flattening of the labiomandibular fold (only on mild to moderate jowls) (**Fig. 14**). Camouflage fat grafting around the labiomandibular area also can markedly help to decrease the deformity. As viewed frontally, prominent labiomandibular areas create a "squared-off" ptotic appearance, contributing to the aged look. This also can be improved

with the aforementioned techniques. The use of a small intraoral incision and subperiosteal dissection of the depressor labii muscle can allow the muscle component of the labiomandibular fold to be released, thereby helping to alleviate the downward-turned corners of the mouth and the prominent mandibular fold as well.[12] Another tool for correcting this deformity is the barbed sutures (usually requiring 2 threads to be placed through the postauricular incision). Barbed sutures can be used in conjunction with suture suspension platysmaplasty for correction of both the midface and brow areas. Finally, an extended skin ellipse with the postauricular skin excision can further correct skin redundancy when prominent jowling is present.

Surgical correction of point 5: mental prominence (chin)

Appropriate chin projection adds tremendously to the overall length and beauty of an aesthetically balanced neck. It also prevents the skin from becoming redundant in the submental area. Cosmetic techniques to augment a deficient or retrussive chin prominence focus primarily around the alloplastic chin implant. The use of sliding genioplasty, with or without wire fixation, is also an

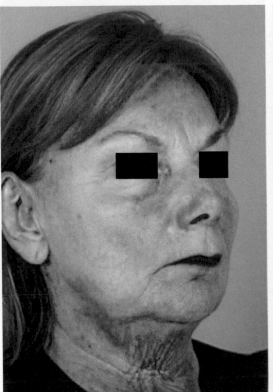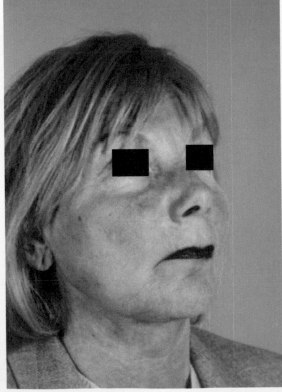

Fig. 14. Surgical correction of Point 4: labiomandibular fold prominence ("jowls").

option, but requires significantly more time, effort, and pain, with more potential complications. Fat grafting to the chin can moderately enhance the chin prominence as well. Long-term fillers have been used with success (**Fig. 15**).

Surgical correction of point 6: anterior neck width

In many patients, the neck width is markedly increased with aging (**Fig. 16**). This increase is mainly attributable to muscle laxity, collapse of the cervical spine, and an increase in subcutaneous and submental fat deposits. The creation of an aesthetically pleasing, thin neck can be accomplished by resection of the redundant midline platysma muscle and reconstitution of the platysma muscle at the midline (see **Fig. 14**). A number of techniques have been described, including midline imbrication,[3] direct excision,[13] or both. It should be noted that oversuctioning or over-resecting of the neck fat can result in a poor final result and can potentially masculanize a feminine neck, especially in the female patient with thin skin.

Postoperative Care

Postoperative care is minimal. Patients are kept on oral pain medications for 3 to 5 days and antibiotics for 1 week. They are instructed to keep their head elevated while sleeping. Dressings and the paper tape are removed after 48 hours. Male patients are advised not to shave for 7 to 10 days after the operation, to avoid trauma to the neck flaps. Patients are instructed to resume activities of daily living in 2 to 3 days and strenuous activity, including exercise, in 3 to 4 weeks.

COMPLICATIONS
Prolonged Tightness of the Neck

It is normal for people to comment about neck tightness, initially, owing to the platysma plication and the suspension suture. If the feeling of tightness persists and is excessive, then this is easily alleviated by a small postauricular incision. With the patient under local anesthesia, identification of the suspension suture, cutting one end, and removing the other end. This will alleviate the tightness, but it will also result in a slight decrease in the definition along the cervicomental angle and mandibular borders.

Wound Dehiscence

Minor complications, such as a small wound dehiscence, have been treated conservatively

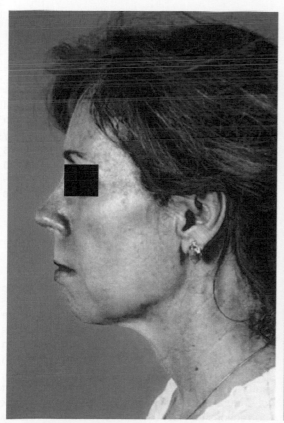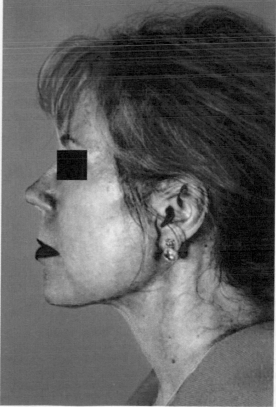

Fig. 15. Surgical correction of Point 5: mental prominence (chin).

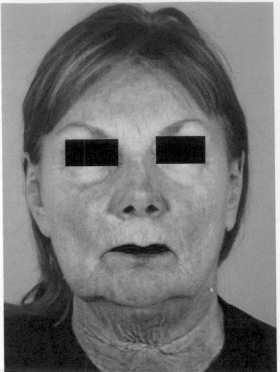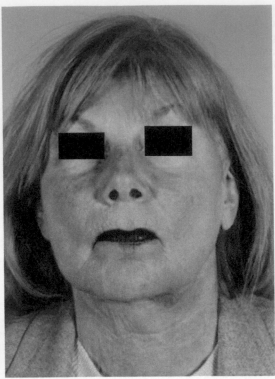

Fig. 16. Surgical correction of Point 6: anterior neck width.

with dressing changes and topical antibiotic ointment, with satisfactory resolution.

Hematoma/Seroma

The rate of hematoma has been less than 1% when fibrin glue sealant is used at the end of the procedure.[14,15] In the case of an immediate postoperative hematoma, drainage is the treatment. If a hematoma forms later, then surgical judgment needs to be exercised. The patient can be taken back to the operating room for drainage, aspirated in the office, or observed, depending on the size of the hematoma and the symptoms. Seromas are usually aspirated in the office.

Prolonged Skin Contracture

Prolonged skin contracture is most likely to happen to the postauricular scar because the superior skin edge of the incision is longer than the inferior skin edge, as a result of the elliptical skin excision. This can result in "bunched-up" skin initially. If the scar is to be kept postauricular, and not extended preauricular, one of the hallmarks of the suture-suspension platysmaplasty technique, then this early result is avoidable by not being overly zealous when excising the postauricular skin. If the scar is hypertrophic, then

Kenalog injections can be used as well as scar massage. Time will also soften the scars.

Asymmetry of the Mouth

Mouth asymmetry could be due to marginal mandibular nerve neuropraxia, edema, or tension on the platysma muscle, creating a temporary depression at the corners of the mouth for patients who have a platysma-depressor labii connection in their muscular anatomy (fewer than I% of all patients). This usually resolves in 2 to 3 months postoperatively.

LONGEVITY OF SUTURE SUSPENSION PLATYSMAPLASTY NECK LIFT

The suture suspension technique is a safe, reproducible technique that allows for a staged rejuvenation of the neck.[6,8] As an alternative for the early rhytidectomy candidate, it produces excellent patient satisfaction outcomes with long-term corrections for most patients. As compared with previously described platysmaplasty techniques, suture suspension platysmaplasty has the benefit of endurance. Publications have shown that neck corrections can last at least 13 years with virtually unchanged aesthetic results (**Fig. 17**).[6]

Pre-Op 6 years 12 years

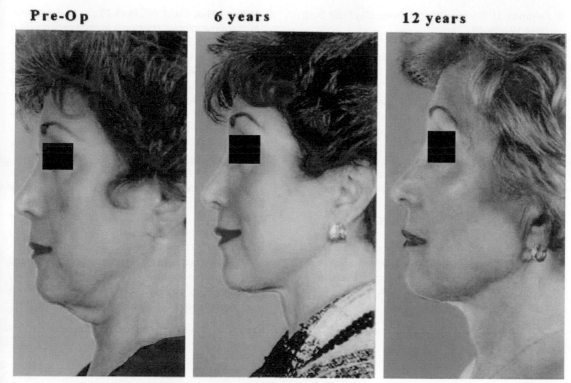

Fig. 17. Long-term outcomes of suture suspension platysmaplasty.

ADVANTAGES OF THE SUTURE SUSPENSION TECHNIQUE FOR NECK REJUVENATION

- Excellent option for male patients who want a nicely contoured neck and jaw without a facelift.
- Quick recovery of 5 to 10 days compared with a facelift.
- Little chance of nerve damage or soft tissue loss, because the neck does not have the abundance of motor nerves that the face has, and the skin undermining is less than in a facelift.
- No preauricular or hair-baring area incisions are involved.
- Can be used during both primary and secondary rhytidectomy for the difficult neck in the obtuse cervicomental angle patients.
- Good option for treating the prolapsed submandibular gland deformity.
- Can be used with certain types of facelift (eg, minilift) to provide a minimally invasive rejuvenation of the face and neck with minimal downtime desired by most patients.

SUMMARY

The suture suspension platysmaplasty neck lift, by creating a permanent artificial "ligament" under the mandible, corrects the deformities of the aging neck with aesthetically pleasing results. In essence, this technique suspends the midline platysma muscle and displaces the lateral platysma muscle under the border of the mandible in a natural way. Fixation of the suture on the mastoid fascia with the appropriate tension is an essential step in this procedure. The tension is adjusted by keeping the head fully rotated and maximally extended to the opposite side of the suture fixation on the mastoid fascia. The "angle loop" modification of the technique further enhances the aesthetic results. Careful analysis of the 6 points of neck rejuvenation and customization of the suture suspension platysmaplasty technique according to these points allows the aesthetic surgeon to fully rejuvenate the neck with a long-lasting result. This technique is simple, safe, and reproducible, with excellent patient satisfaction outcomes.

REFERENCES

1. Ellenbogen R, Karlin JV. Visual criteria for success in restoring the youthful neck. Plast Reconstr Surg 1980;66:826–37.
2. Guerrero-Santos J, Espaillat L, Morales F. Muscular lift in cervical rhytidoplasty. Plast Reconstr Surg 1974;54:127–30.

3. Feldman JJ. Corset platysmaplasty. Clin Plast Surg 1992;19:369–82.

4. Conrad K, Chapnik JS, Reifen E. E-PTFE (Gore-Tex) suspension cervical facial rhytidectomy. Arch Otolaryngol Head Neck Surg 1993;119:694–8.

5. Giampapa VC, Di Bernardo BE. Neck recontouring with suture suspension and liposuction: an alternative for the early rhytidectomy candidate. Aesthetic Plast Surg 1995;19:217–23.

6. Giampapa V, Bitzos I, Ramirez O, et al. Long-term results of suture suspension platysmaplasty for neck rejuvenation: a 13-year follow-up evaluation. Aesthetic Plast Surg 2005;29:332–40.

7. Nahai F. Reconsidering neck suspension sutures. Aesthet Surg J 2004;24:365–7.

8. Giampapa V, Bitzos I, Ramirez O, et al. Suture suspension platysmaplasty for neck rejuvenation revisited: technical fine points for improving outcomes. Aesthetic Plast Surg 2005;29:341–50 [discussion: 351–2].

9. Millard DR Jr, Garst WP, Beck RL, et al. Submental and submandibular lipectomy in conjunction with a face lift, in the male or female. Plast Reconstr Surg 1972;49:385–91.

10. Mesa JM, Vasconez LO. Face and neck-lifts under local anesthesia with neither IV sedation nor general anesthesia. American Association of Plastic Surgeons 2013 Annual Meeting & Symposia. New Orleans (LA), 2013.

11. Ramirez OM. Cervicoplasty: nonexcisional anterior approach. Plast Reconstr Surg 1997;99:1576–85.

12. Hoefflin SM. Anatomy of the platysma and lip depressor muscles. A simplified mnemonic approach. Dermatol Surg 1998;24:1225–31.

13. Henderson J, O'Neill T, Logan A. Direct anterior neck skin excision for cervicomental laxity. Aesthetic Plast Surg 2010;34:299–305.

14. Ellis DA, Pelausa EO. Fibrin glue in facial plastic and reconstructive surgery. J Otolaryngol 1988;17:74–7.

15. Giampapa VC, Bitar GJ. Use of fibrin sealant in neck contouring. Aesthet Surg J 2002;22:519–25.

Rejuvenation of the Aging Neck
40 Years Experience

Brunno Ristow, MD, FACS

KEYWORDS

- Neck lift • Neck lift technique • Neck lift sequelae • Neck lift complications • Neck rejuvenation

KEY POINTS

- The neck is divided into 2 defined segments: (1) the submental, submandibular region, and (2) the region of the neck proper, which includes the structures caudally to this imaginary line.
- The understanding of neck rejuvenation depends entirely on 2 different factors. Alone, neither will produce a good neck. Combine both, and an excellent result is consistently achieved.
- The correction of laxity of tissues in the submental area needs direct surgery in this region and the hammock effect, produced by the bilateral elevation of the midface lift. Only with both can the rejuvenation of this region be achieved.

Editor Commentary: My friendship with Bruno Ristow exceeds 35 years, and I was delighted when he accepted my invitation to contribute to this publication. He followed the questions posed to him and presents a logical template for rejuvenating the neck. He makes the important point of proper rotation of the SMAS/platysma flap following partial transection of the platysma at the level of the cricoid carti-lage. His admonition to wait up to 1 year before considering revising the neck is important to consider, because many small issues resolve themselves; larger issues require maturation of the soft tissue (similar to waiting 1 year before performing a secondary rhinoplasty.)

INTRODUCTION

When the editor of this issue asked me to share my experience and the concluding thoughts resulting from my nearly 40 years of performing neck rejuvenation, I promptly and happily accepted the invitation. The reasons are simply based on experience; to me the issues have logical and direct answers based on facts. I was prompted with a series of questions to address. However, before I address the questions, I want to emphasize that the understanding of neck rejuvenation depends entirely on 2 different factors. Neither will produce a good neck alone. Combine both, and an excellent result is consistently achieved.

If a fine line is drawn from the jaw neck angle to the earlobe (**Fig. 1**), the neck is divided into 2 defined segments:

1. The submental, submandibular region
2. The region of the neck proper, which includes the structures caudally to this imaginary line

The correction of laxity of tissues in the submental area, need, aside from the direct surgery in this region, needs the hammock effect, produced by the bilateral elevation of the midface lift. Only then, can the rejuvenation of this region be achieved. The effect of the superficial musculo-aponeurotic system (SMAS) elevation on the right and left midface, gives a strong

California Pacific Medical Center, San Francisco, CA
E-mail address: info@brunnoristow.com

Clin Plastic Surg 41 (2014) 125–129
http://dx.doi.org/10.1016/j.cps.2013.09.004
0094-1298/14/$ – see front matter © 2014 Elsevier Inc. All rights reserved.

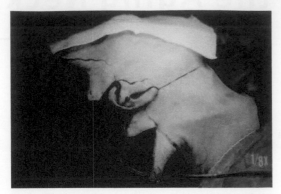

Fig. 1. Dividing the neck into aesthetic units and skin redraping.

sling effect to the tissues in the submental region, appropriately described as the hammock effect.

Now, to address specific questions.

WHAT INCISION(S) DO YOU TYPICALLY USE IN THE THIN NECK AND THE HEAVY NECK IN BOTH YOUNG AND OLDER PATIENTS?

Younger and older patients will receive very similar incisions. In the older ones, necessarily the occipital incision has to be longer. Only young patients,

with localized submental fat and no plastymal bands, are treated with–occipital incision (**Figs. 2** and **3**).

WHAT ARE YOUR INDICATIONS FOR LIMITING YOUR ACCESS INCISIONS TO THE SUBMENTAL AREA OR THE LATERAL APPROACH? IN WHICH CASES DO YOU USE BOTH INCISIONS?

In a still youthful neck with good skin texture and only localized submental fat, a simple submental incision, 3.5 cm long, located 1 cm below the submental crease, is sufficient for effective treatment. The submental crease is released, as are the attachments to the depressors of the lip bilaterally. Silverglyde Bipolar forceps (Stryker Corporation/ Kalamazoo, MI) is the only safe approach to hemeostasis over the depressor anguli oris. The localized fat is taken out in progressive layers until the platysma muscle is exposed. If necessary, 1, 2, or 3 sutures between the thyroid cartilage and the symphisis of mentum are placed to assure an attractive jaw/neck angle. A Porex (Porex Medical Products/Ontario, CA) (1-800-521-7321, ECO-043-02) drain is placed and the incision closed, everting its edges, with a 6-0 suture.

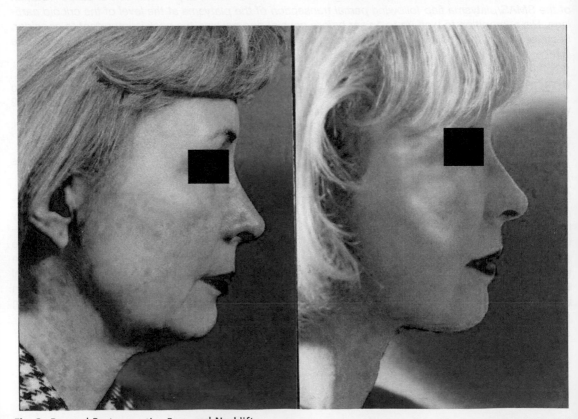

Fig. 2. Pre and Post-operative Face and Necklift.

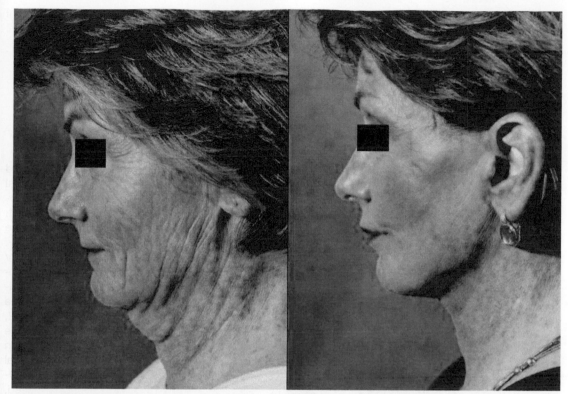

Fig. 3. Pre and Post-operative Face and Necklift.

Most patients who need their neck rejuvenated need a retroauricular occipital incision. Whenever the structures (skin/muscle) are aged, this redraping becomes necessary. The vectors of redraping allow for little variation. Generally, they are at 90° from the neck (see **Fig. 1**).

WHAT IS YOUR APPROACH TO DEFATTING THE NECK? WHICH FATTY LAYERS DO YOU RESECT (IE, SUBCUTANEOUS, INTERPLATYSMAL, SUBPLATYSMAL FAT)? WHAT ROLE DOES LIPOSUCTION PLAY IN YOUR TECHNIQUE, EITHER ALONE OR IN COMBINATION WITH OPEN TECHNIQUES?

I choose to elevate the skin of the neck with the appropriate final thickness of the subcutaneous fat. I gauge this by feeling the dissecting scissors on my right hand and my fifth finger on my left hand to feel the thickness of the flap of the skin being elevated. I find this method accurate and equally precise as transillumination. After the final positioning of the platysma, with the sling to the occipital region (or the small flap described by Tord Skoog[1]), I defat the layer overlaying the platysma (**Fig. 4**). (Transillumination is used to evaluate the uniform thickness

of the flaps at the end of the procedure, just prior to closure.)

HOW DOES THE PRESENCE OF VISIBLE PLATYSMA MUSCLE BANDS ALTER YOUR APPROACH? DO YOU UNDERMINE, PLICATE, TRANSECT, PARTIALLY RESECT, OR BACKCUT PLATYSMAL MUSCLE BANDS?

Visible platysma muscle bands are always treated. The central strip of platysma is removed; submental fat is grasped with a brown forceps and resected. This leaves platysmal edges on both sides, generally separated by 2 cm. These edges are sutured together in the midline; usually 3 sutures with inverted knots of 3-0 nylon between the thyroid cartilage and the symphisis of the mentum are sufficient. The continuity of the bands is interrupted at the level of the cricoid cartilage, for 2.5 cm in each direction, with a triangle of the muscle removed.

Laterally, I also routinely partially divide the platysma muscle. I follow the anterior border of the sternocleidomastoideus muscle, approximately 5 cm (or more if necessary) toward the direction of the cricoid cartilage. The platysma/SMAS flap resulting from the midface dissection is then

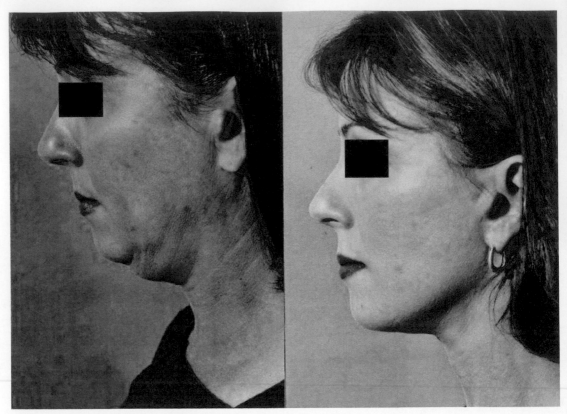

Fig. 4. Pre and Post-operative Face and Necklift.

transposed to the retroauricular/occipital region. I do not plicate the platysma, as I suspect this may contribute to the later formation of recurring bands.

DISCUSS SUBMAXILLARY GLAND REDUCTION

A good platysma/SMAS sling, with the midline anchoring sutures, provides significant subman-dibular support. Given reported complications and drawbacks (eg, dry mouth, halitosis, fistulas, and rare nerve injuries), I have not engaged in the partial resection of the glands. Also, after expla-nation to prospective patients of the issues involved, I have observed that patients will not accept this procedure.

DO YOU PARTIALLY RESECT THE ANTERIOR BELLIES OF THE DIGASTRIC MUSCLES?

Yes, I do partially resect the anterior bellies of the digastric, but only if they are responsible for extra bulk. I electrocoagulate the excessive volume.

DO YOU FEEL THERE IS A NEED TO DRAIN NECKS?

Yes, I drain all necks. A major and difficult problem is to have any remaining blood after surgery. Avoidance of this complication is of paramount importance.

DO YOU USE FIBRIN GLUE IN THE NECK?

No, I do not use fibrin glue in the neck. I am con-cerned about the manufacturers' disclaimers of possible transmission of disease.

BRIEFLY MENTION EXPECTED SEQUELAE OF YOUR TECHNIQUE AND COMPLICATIONS THAT YOU HAVE OBSERVED AND HOW YOU TREATED THEM

Collections of undrained blood and rare banding of the platysma are difficult issues. They require time for reabsorption, patience, good relations with one's patients, and, extremely rarely, excision of the offending band. Lesser issues may respond to BOTOX and judicious injections of diluted Triamcinolone Acetonide.

MENTION YOUR TIMING FOR ANY REVISIONS OF A NECK LIFT

I would wait 1 year if it all possible. Revisions, however, have practically not existed, following the technical precautions aforementioned. Unfortunately, I have seen very poor results from surgery done elsewhere, frequently, not amendable to improvement. Too much fat removed from the subcutaneous layer and the excessive electrocoagulation are often the culprits.

REFERENCE

1. Tord Skoog I. Plastic Surgery - New Methods and Refinement. Stockholm, Sweden: Almquist & Wiksell International; 1974.

Serendipity in Ultimate Neck Lift Correction

Richard Ellenbogen, MD, FACS*, Urmen Desai, MD, MPH

KEYWORDS

- Neck lift • Fat grafting • Liposuction

KEY POINTS

- By performing a necklift by this technique many pearl size pieces of fat were created. These "pearl fat grafts" were placed in various folds and depression of the face as filler.
- The fat removed from the neck was grafted through incisions and tunnels in the face.
- Three principals in the technique include removal of fat to the inferior mandibular border, tighten the loose muscle to create a youthful neck and allow the skin to redrape by its own elasticity.

Editor Commentary: It is more than 30 years since Richard Ellenbogen described the essential visual criteria for restoring a youthful neck. I encourage readers to keep these criteria in mind as they read the other articles in this coverage of neck lift. In this article, Richard describes how his technique for rejuvenating the neck has evolved, always setting the goals of a happy patient, a predictable result, and minimizing the risk of complications by keeping it simple.

After a visit to Bruce Connell in 1975, I (Dr Ellenbogen) realized I had seen the ultimate answer to neck correction in facelifts—the treatment of the muscles, the removal of fat both superficial and deep, and the skin tightening. Dr Connell's patients were older than mine, as a rule, and, as a young plastic surgeon, I devised a neck-only lift using his principles.

These consisted of

- Submental incision
- Removal of all fat inferior to the mandibular border
- Closing the platysmas at the midline
- Cutting the platysma at the level of the hyoid
- Exercising great care with the proximity to the marginal mandibular nerve, and
- Allowing the natural elasticity of the skin to retract over the new framework

Dr Connell had never done the neck at this time as an isolated procedure. When I published in *Plastic and Reconstructive Surgery* in 1980,[1] I entertained doctors from around the globe, demonstrating the technique for a procedure that I did not think deserved any special recognition because Guerrosantos had already done it.

I had, at the termination of each neck lift, a pile of small pieces of fat removed from the neck and began placing them in tunnels thru the nostril into the nasolabial folds and in the lips and cheekbones. I researched the world's literature on fat grafting and noted that "pearl fat grafts"[2] were done in the early 1900s. This fat grafting was 7 years before the liposuction task force returned from France. The extraction of fat by cannula was not yet devised in America.

My neck article was published in 1980, 2 years after submission to an academic journal. My rediscovery of fat grafting was submitted 4 times over 4 years to an academic journal and returned with the criticism, "grafted fat doesn't last." It was ultimately published in *Annals of Plastic Surgery* in 1984[2] after many lectures at various professional societies.[3] Sydney Coleman, while a resident in San Francisco, attended my lecture and spread the word that fat does graft and remain. In the

Beverly Hills Body, 2080 Century Park East, Suite #501, Los Angeles, CA 90067, USA
* Corresponding author.
E-mail address: richinmind@aol.com

Clin Plastic Surg 41 (2014) 131–138
http://dx.doi.org/10.1016/j.cps.2013.09.009
0094-1298/14/$ – see front matter © 2014 Elsevier Inc. All rights reserved.

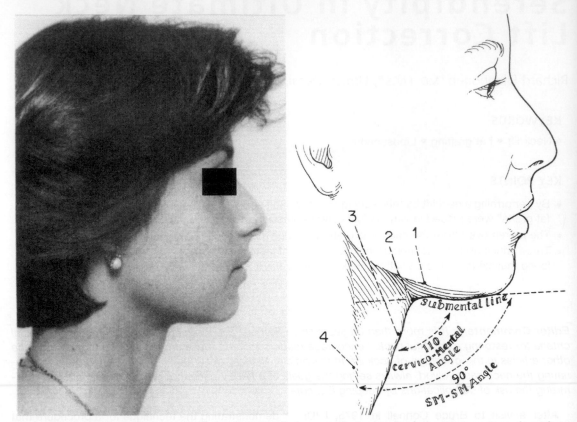

Fig. 1. The youthful neck has 5 criteria: (1) distinct inferior mandibular border from mentum to angle with no jowl over hang, (2) subhyoid depression (without this slight recess below the apex of the cervicomental angle the neck neck does not appear thin and long), (3) visible thyroid cartilage, (4) visible anterior border of sterno-cleidomastoid muscle form the mastoid to the sternum, and (5) cervicomental angle between 105° and 120°. (*From* Ellenbogen R. Free autogenous pearl fat grafts in the face–a preliminary report of a rediscovered technique. Ann Plast Surg 1986;16(3):179–94; with permission.)

performance of my neck lift, fat grafting was redis-covered serendipitously.

WHY IS A NECK LIFT LIKE A KISS?

Dr Ruth once said, "When you kiss do you do it to please your partner or please yourself?" A neck lift is very much like this. Of course, the patient must be pleased foremost but many physicians try too hard and use extraneous or possibly unnecessary techniques when possibly not necessary (gland excision, digastric excision, platysma cutting or excision, and postauricular excision).

Another kiss analogy is KISS—*keep it* simple *stupid*. Avoid variations with higher complications and prolonged recovery. My techniques and thou-sands of neck lifts follow that principle.

SURGICAL APPROACH

My approach, and this is a simplified version of my present approach, was learned after many favor-able and less than favorable results

- I almost universally use a submental incision of approximately 2–3 cm back from the infe-rior mandibular border at the midline.
- I do not use tumescent anesthesia. It seems to cloud the muscle fat border colors and makes excision or the fat more difficult.
- I inject 20 mL of 1/200,000, 0.5% lidocaine, and listen to country music for 20 minutes.
- I dissect the fat from the skin and scrupu-lously remove the fat superficial to the platysma below the inferior mandibular border.
- In a fat or heavy neck, I separate the platys-mas at the midline and remove subplatysma fat, cauterizing well all bleeders.
- I see no reason to ever remove the digastrics. I remove as far as I can posteriorly by direct vision.
- I make a small incision behind the earlobe and, with a 3-mm cannula, suction the fat at the angle of the mandible I could not see from the midline incision and liposuction the

borders of the fat excision inferiorly to feather all edges.

- I close the platysma with buried 4-0 nylon.
- I rarely remove an anterior platysma border unless the platysma is flaccid on closure.

- I insert a 3-mm suction drain in each postauricular liposuction cannula hole.
- The incision under the neck is closed subcuticularly and a light compression dressing is used for 24 hours.

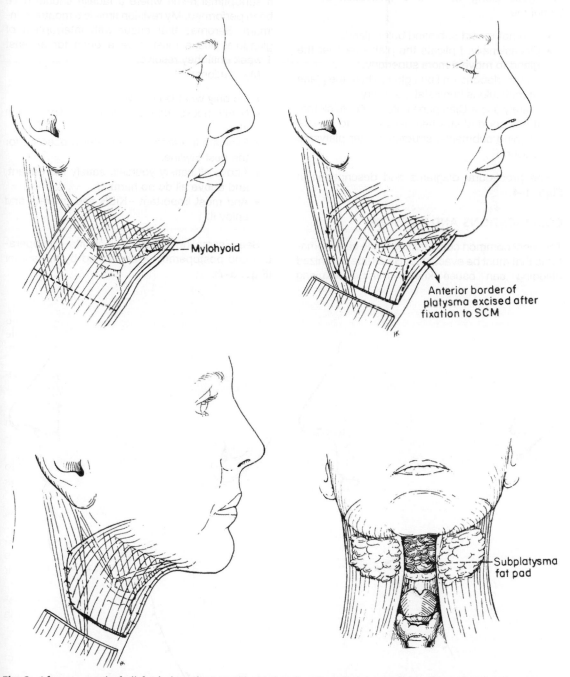

Fig. 2. After removal of all fat below the mandibular border, the subplatysma fat pad is evaluated for removal. The posterior border of the platysma is sutured to the sternocleidomastoid and the platysma transected and the anterior border is excised. The midline is closed with 4-0 nylon. (*From* Ellenbogen R. Free autogenous pearl fat grafts in the face–a preliminary report of a rediscovered technique. Ann Plast Surg 1986;16(3):179–94; with permission.)

- I use a postauricular skin and platysma tightening incision only rarely, when it is obvious that lax skin must be tightened—usually in the older thin neck.

I have simplified the description of my technique that goes along with the simplification of my technique:

- I do not resect submandibular gland.
- Occasionally, I plicate the platysma over the gland to move it more superiorly.
- I never depend on fibrin glue to take the place of meticulous hemostatic surgery.
- I rarely use a Giampapa stitch, but I think that it is a good idea, when necessary, to elevate sagging submental structures after platysma closure.

See procedural diagrams and descriptions in **Figs. 1–4**.

COMPLICATIONS AND REVISIONS

The most common complication is the early hematoma that must be evacuated. Small late organized bleeding can cause knotty bumps requiring monthly dilute triamcinolone (Kenalog) shots. Failure to excise all fat inferior to the jawline may require a local liposuction procedure. Occasionally, the platysma closure forms a tight band that responds to excision. For me, the most troubling complication is misjudging the neck and getting a suboptimal result where a facelift should have been performed. My revision time is 6 months minimum. Seromas that occur with interruption of glandular tissue must have a drain for at least 1 week until they resolve.

My cautions:

- Do only what is necessary.
- Many necks can be done by liposuction alone.
- Evaluate if a facelift is a better procedure for the best jawline.
- Above all satisfy yourself, satisfy the patient, and above all do no harm.
- And most important—KISS and operate and enjoy it.

See a sampling of patient neck lifts—preoperative and postoperative—performed by the author (**Figs. 5–7**).

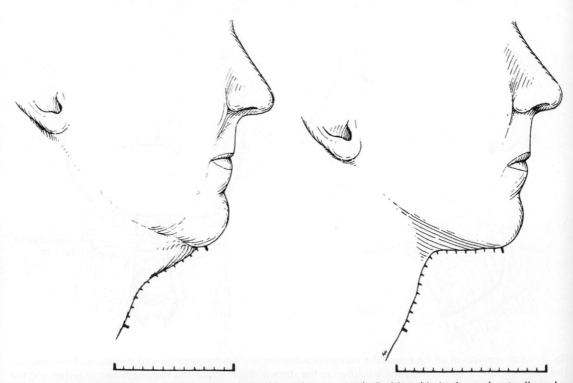

Fig. 3. Heavy neck patients actually have too little skin rather too much. Excising skin in the neck actually makes the neck heavier. (*From* Ellenbogen R. Free autogenous pearl fat grafts in the face–a preliminary report of a rediscovered technique. Ann Plast Surg 1986;16(3):179–94; with permission.)

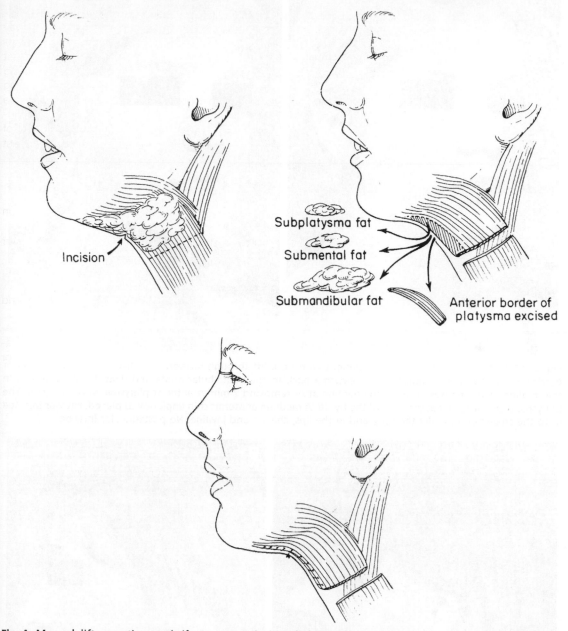

Incision

Subplatysma fat

Submental fat

Submandibular fat

Anterior border of platysma excised

Fig. 4. My neck lift operation rarely if ever uses an incision behind the ear. Through a 2–3 cm incision made 3 cm back from the mentum, the fat superficial to the platysma and overlapping the mandibular border is removed under direct vision. The platysma is transected and subplatysma fat is evaluated. Anterior border of platysma is excised and platysma borders are closed with 4-0 nylon. (*From* Ellenbogen R. Free autogenous pearl fat grafts in the face–a preliminary report of a rediscovered technique. Ann Plast Surg 1986;16(3):179–94; with permission.)

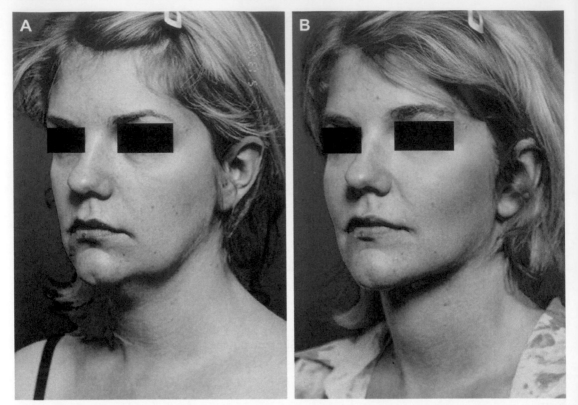

Fig. 5. (*A–B*) A 36-year-old weight loss patient with neck lift through incision 3 cm from mandibular anterior border. Fat was removed superficial to platysma back to the mandibular angle and deep to the platysma in the midline. Platysma was closed in the midline after removing 7 mm of anterior platysma with 4-0 nylon. The platysma was transected at the level of the hyoid. A medium anatomic chin implant was placed. Fat was injected in to the cheekbones, under the eyes, and in the lips, cheeks, and jawline. No postauricular incision.

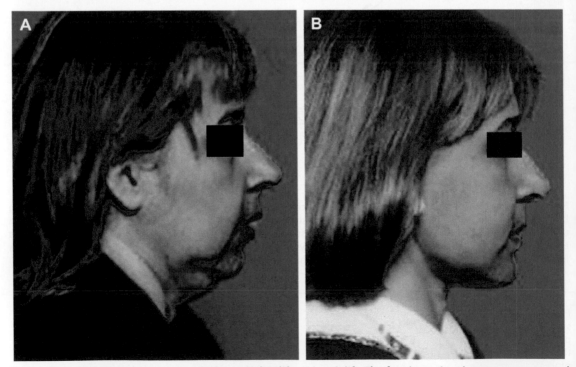

Fig. 6. (*A–B*) A 48-year-old woman with skin only facelift and neck lift. The fat above the platysma was removed under direct vision. The fat below the platysma was removed to expose the digastric. The platysma was transected at the level of the hyoid; 7 mm of medial platysma was removed from either side and closed in the midline with 4-0 nylon. The platysma was sutured to the sternocleidomastoid posteriorly. Fat was injected in to the cheekbones, cheeks, and under eyes. A 7-mm anatomic chin implant was used.

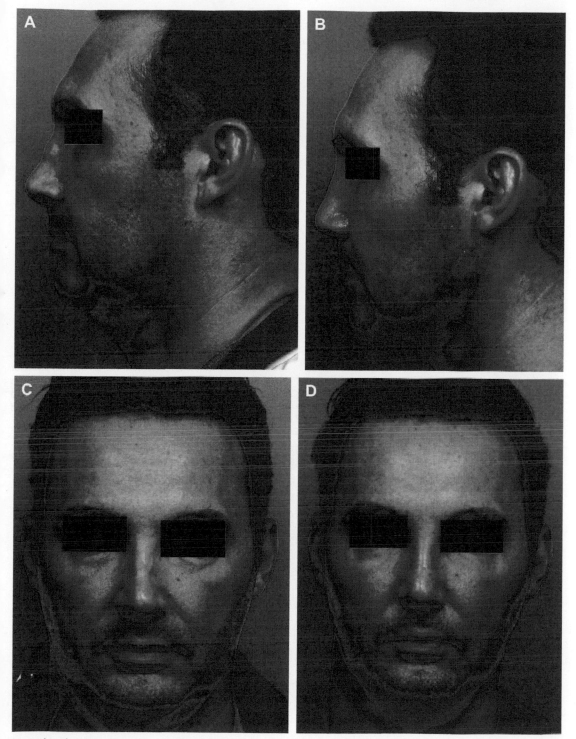

Fig. 7. (*A–D*) A 44-year-old man refuses facelift. The entire procedure was performed through a submental incision approximately 3 cm. All fat was removed superficial to platysma and inferior to the mandibular border. Subplatysma fat was removed to the digastric; 1 cm of anterior platysma was removed and the platysma transected at the level of the hyoid. The platysma was closed pants over vest in the midline with 4-0 nylon. Drains were left over night.

REFERENCES

1. Ellenbogen R, Karlin JV. Visual criteria for success in restoring the youthful neck. Plast Reconstr Surg 1980; 66(6):826–37.

2. Ellenbogen R. Free autogenous pearl fat grafts in the face- a preliminary report of a rediscovered technique. Ann Plast Surg 1986;16(3):179–94.

3. Presented California Plastic Surgery Society. Lahaina, Hawaii, 1984.

Neck Lift Technique
The Lifestyle Lift

Malcolm D. Paul, MD, FACS

KEYWORDS

- Lifestyle lift • Level 1 anesthesia • Sequelae • Complications

KEY POINTS

- A full range of facial aesthetic surgical procedures can be performed safely and quickly with Level 1 anesthesia, avoiding the risks associated with general anesthesia.
- More than 95% of all of the varieties of aging neck pathology require an open submental approach for evaluation and treatment of fat deposits and varying patterns of platysma muscle bands.
- Draining all necklifts seems to reduce the incidence of small blood and serum collections.
- Sequelae and complications with facelifts performed under Level 1 anesthesia are acceptable and can be managed based upon the clinical findings.

Editor Commentary: *This chapter describes the author's current techniqeue for rejuvenating the aging neck using only oral sedation, oral analgesia, and local infiltrative anesthesia. All of the anatomic findings in aging necks from simple submental mild lipodystrophy without skin excell to obtuse cervical/mental angles with excessive fat in all of the compartments of the neck can be safely managed with this technique. Patient risks are minimized by avoiding general anesthesia with its' possible sequelae and complications including, but not limited to: emergence related hypertension, respiratory compromise, DVTs, and pulmonary emboli. Not having to work around a nasal or oral tube is an added advantage. The author has safely utilized this approach in patients aged 45–95, and, contrary to the comments of the critics of the Lifestyle Lift, the range of procedures offered and the results obtained by Lifestyle Lift surgeons nationwide are as good as any I have seen in viewing techniques and results worldwide for over 38 years.*

MANAGING AGING NECKS UNDER LEVEL 1 ANESTHESIA: THE LIFESTYLE LIFT

There are many surgical solutions for the aging neck, from closed liposuction, closed or minimal access thread suspension, to open minimally and moderately aggressive approaches with oral sedation and analgesia or with general anesthesia. I am comfortable with a range of procedures, all performed under local anesthesia with oral sedation and analgesia, to provide a safe, efficient, reproducible, necklift that addresses all the components of the aging neck from the cutaneous envelope to the deep fat compartments (**Figs. 1–3**).

My responses to questions asked for managing different types of necks are as follows.

WHAT INCISION(S) DO YOU TYPICALLY USE IN THE THIN NECK AND THE HEAVY NECK IN BOTH YOUNG AND OLDER PATIENTS?
Thin Neck

A thin neck may only require a small submental incision for minimal liposuction access or a wider incision to address platysmal bands. However, frequently, platysma muscle bands become visible after the overlying fat has been suctioned or resected and the incision needs to be lengthened to allow access for midline muscle suturing. Frequently, a periauricular incision is required as well for drain placement and for skin redraping. These methods are more commonly used in younger patients and rarely in older patients who demonstrate a tight skin envelope. Most

Aesthetic and Plastic Surgery Institute, University of California, Irvine, 1401 Avocado Avenue, Suite 610, Newport Beach, CA 92660, USA
E-mail address: mpaulmd@hotmail.com

Clin Plastic Surg 41 (2014) 139–143
http://dx.doi.org/10.1016/j.cps.2013.09.010
0094-1298/14/$ – see front matter © 2014 Elsevier Inc. All rights reserved.

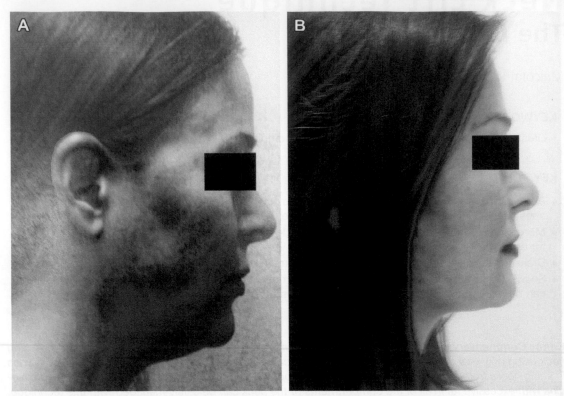

Fig. 1. A 45-year-old woman underwent lifestyle lift and open, blind, temporal lift: (*A*) before, (*B*) after the operation.

commonly, a short incision or traditional face and necklift incision is required to adequately treat the aging neck.

Thick Neck

A thick skin neck requires both incisions unless there are no significant platysma muscle bands and the skin quality is good, which may allow liposuction alone from small puncture points below the ear lobule and in the submental area. This is seen in patients of all ages. Again, a short incision or a traditional face and necklift incision is required to treat the relevant deformities.

WHAT IS YOUR APPROACH TO DEFATTING THE HEAVY NECK? WHICH FATTY LAYERS DO YOU RESECT (SUBCUTANEOUS, INTERPLATYSMAL, SUBPLATYSMAL FAT)?

Closed liposuction is effective in heavy necks, however, this only addresses fat that is anterior to the platysma muscles. Often, interplatysmal and subplatysmal fat must be contoured, but not overresected; overresection may be extremely difficult to correct.

HOW DOES THE PRESENCE OF VISIBLE PLATYSMA MUSCLE BANDS ALTER YOUR APPROACH? DO YOU UNDERMINE, PLICATE, TRANSECT, PARTIALLY RESECT PLATYSMAL MUSCLE BANDS?
Tighten Platysmal Bands

I have tried to merely tighten platysmal bands from the lateral approach, but I have not succeeded in preventing recurrence of these bands, most often in patients who exhibit bands from the mandible to the clavicles.

Open Approach

I open in more than 95% of all necks. I begin with closed pretunneling and liposuction in heavier necks followed by open evaluation and contouring of the fat compartments. The platysma muscle bands are identified, undermined, and united with barbed sutures followed by placement of interrupted absorbable sutures (polylactic acid derived). A backcut of the platysma muscles for about 2 cm is performed in all cases where bands are full length from the mandible to the clavicles.

The lateral approach is joined with the midline approach, first with sequential tunnelers followed by flap dissection. Lateral platysmaplasty is routinely

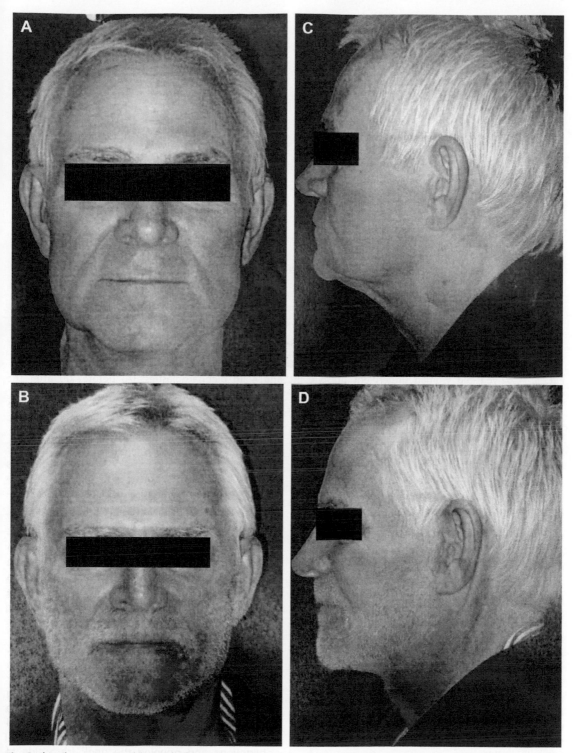

Fig. 2. (*A, C*). A 60-year-old man before lifestyle lift: (*A*) front view; (*C*) side view. (*B, D*) A 60-year-old man after lifestyle lift: (*B*) front view; (*D*) side view.

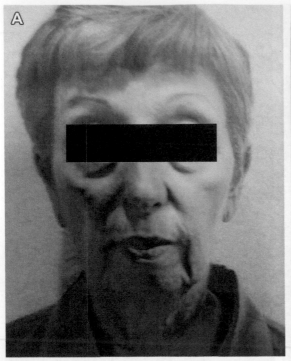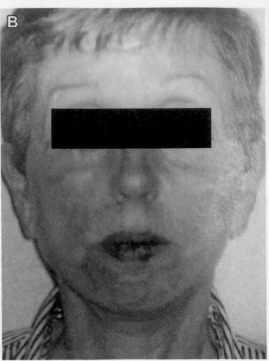

Fig. 3. A 62-year-old woman underwent lifestyle lift and 4 lid blepharoplasties: (*A*) before, (*B*) after the operation.

added with barbed sutures anchored to the Lore fascia. The neck skin is redraped carefully and resected in a direction that avoids traction lines that are not aligned with the relaxed skin tension lines.

DISCUSS SUBMAXILLARY GLAND REDUCTION

I have not performed submaxillary gland resection and I prefer to suspend the gland under the mandibular border.

DO YOU PARTIALLY RESECT THE ANTERIOR BELLIES OF THE DIGASTRIC MUSCLES?

No, I do not perform this maneuver and, although I have identified the anterior bellies of the digastric muscles as detractors from an ideal neck contour, I have seen overly sculpted necks that are nearly impossible to correct when these muscles have been partially resected. I have seen excellent neck contouring with this maneuver, but an undesirable result that I could not correct deters me from doing this.

DO YOU THINK THERE IS A NEED TO DRAIN NECKS?

I drain every neck and I think that these drains need to be in place for at least 2 days to allow

for adherence of the dissected neck flap. Collections of blood and serum in the neck can be difficult to resolve without insertion of a drain after the fact or repeated aspirations. Indurated necks take a long time to soften and patients are unhappy with the need for frequent visits, aspirations, compressive dressings, and so forth.

DO YOU USE FIBRIN GLUE IN THE NECK?

I used fibrin glue several years ago, but I abandoned it when I had to treat small pseudobursa that formed from the pooling of the glue. Perhaps I will revisit this tool in heavy necks and in all men who are more prone to hematoma and seroma formations.

SEQUELAE AND COMPLICATIONS OF NECK LIFT

More aggressive procedures may result in more frequent sequelae and complications. Most patients want a rapid return to their work and social obligations and opening the neck from side to side arguably provides a greater opportunity for hematoma, seroma, chronic induration, contour irregularities, and in smokers, an increased risk of skin necrosis. Using sequential dilators to undermine the skin of the neck allows for the preservation of fasciocutaneous perforators that nourish a flap that has been compromised by the effects of smoking on the microcirculation of the flap. Minor contour irregularities improve with time, massage, compression, and, where indicated, judicious injections of a small concentration of triamcinolone. I do not believe that large hematomas can be rinsed out. The result of not opening a neck that displays a large hematoma is an agonizing period of healing for the patient with a predictable poor outcome that frequently requires open revision. Small collections behind the ear can be evacuated and a drain inserted.

Recurrent skin laxity is most often the result of inadequate undermining or a failure to observe the quality of the skin before the procedure. Postoperative skin tightening can be achieved with noninvasive or minimally invasive energy-based solutions, thereby avoiding the need to reopen the neck in some cases. Residual fat pockets can be addressed with minimally invasive devices (radiotherapy, ultrasound, and laser-based energies) or with small-cannula closed liposuction.

Recurrent platysma muscle bands can be treated by the following:

1. Closed myotomy with a wire or a braided suture to saw through the band(s)
2. Repeat botulinum toxin injections separated by about 1 cm along each band, but not behind the band that may cause a problem with deglutition
3. Reopening the neck no sooner than 9 to 12 months postoperatively unless only minor skin redraping or neck contouring with fat resection and/or platysma muscle midline suturing is required

Unfavorable scarring related to a propensity to florid scar formation due to an ethnic or social habit (seen in smokers and in patients of color) can be treated with topical scar therapy medications, pressure dressings, lasers, triamcinalone injections, scar revisions, and in the case of hypertrophic or keloid scars, scar excision, closure, and immediate low-dose radiation therapy.

Over the past year, regardless of the complexity of the problems that I have to address in the aging neck, I am comfortable with my ability to perform these procedures under level 1 anesthesia (oral sedation and analgesia), as an outpatient, without an overnight stay, with immediate ambulation, and adequate postoperative monitoring of each patient's recovery. Although I have not reviewed all my cases, I believe that my rate of sequelae and complications is certainly no greater and might be less with this approach to surgical correction of the aging neck.

Index

Note: Page numbers of article titles are in **boldface** type.

Clin Plastic Surg 41 (2014) 145–147
http://dx.doi.org/10.1016/S0094-1298(13)00132-6
0094-1298/14/$ – see front matter © 2014 Elsevier Inc. All rights reserved.

plasticsurgery.theclinics.com

Printed and bound by CPI Group (UK) Ltd, Croydon, CR0 4YY

03/10/2024

01040309-0011